T0331274

Livestock Ration Formulation for Dairy Cattle and Buffalo

Livestock Ration Formulation for Dairy Cattle and Buffalo

Ravinder Singh Kuntal
Assistant Professor, Department of Mathematics, Faculty of Engineering and Technology, Jain (Deemed-to-Be) University, Bengaluru, Karnataka, India

Radha Gupta
Department of Mathematics, Dayananda Sagar College of Engineering, Bengaluru, Karnataka, India

D. Rajendran
ICAR-National Institute of Animal Nutrition and Physiology, Bengaluru, Karnataka, India

Vishal Patil
Department of Mathematics, Faculty of Engineering and Technology, Jain (Deemed-to-be) University, Bengaluru, Karnataka, India

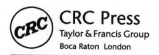

CRC Press
Taylor & Francis Group
Boca Raton London

CRC Press is an imprint of the
Taylor & Francis Group, an **informa** business

MATLAB® is a trademark of The MathWorks, Inc. and is used with permission. The MathWorks does not warrant the accuracy of the text or exercises in this book. This book's use or discussion of MATLAB® software or related products does not constitute endorsement or sponsorship by The MathWorks of a particular pedagogical approach or particular use of the MATLAB® software.

First edition published 2022
by CRC Press
6000 Broken Sound Parkway NW, Suite 300, Boca Raton, FL 33487–2742

and by CRC Press
2 Park Square, Milton Park, Abingdon, Oxon, OX14 4RN

© 2022 Ravinder Singh Kuntal, Radha Gupta, Rajendran D and Vishal Patil

CRC Press is an imprint of Taylor & Francis Group, LLC

Library of Congress Cataloging-in-Publication Data
Names: Singh Kuntal, Ravinder, author. | Gupta, Radha, 1970– author. |
    Rajendran, D., author. | Patil, Vishal, author.
Title: Livestock ration formulation for dairy cattle and buffalo /
    Ravinder Singh Kuntal, Radha Gupta, Rajendran D, Vishal Patil.
Description: First edition | Boca Raton, FL : CRC Press, 2022. |
    Includes bibliographical references and index.
Identifiers: LCCN 2021048758 | ISBN 9781032137476 (hardback) |
    ISBN 9781032139678 (paperback) | ISBN 9781003231714 (ebook)
Subjects: LCSH: Dairy cattle—Feeds and feeding. | Buffaloes—Feeds and
    feeding. | Dairy farming. | Animal nutrition. | Handbooks and manuals.
Classification: LCC SF95 .S564 2022 | DDC 636.08/52—dc23/eng/20211122
LC record available at https://lccn.loc.gov/2021048758

ISBN: 978-1-032-13747-6 (hbk)
ISBN: 978-1-032-13967-8 (pbk)
ISBN: 978-1-003-23171-4 (ebk)

DOI: 10.1201/9781003231714

Typeset in Times
by Apex CoVantage, LLC

This book is dedicated to the memory of my beloved father

Late Warrant Officer R.L Verma (1956–1999)

&

To my mother

Smt. Premvati Devi Verma

You are profoundly appreciated for your unflinching

commitment to the pursuit of my career

And also, to my son, Vivaan

This book was written when you were separated from me,

and I just want to tell you that I love you so much.

Contents

Tables

Figures

Preface

Optimization is one of the important areas of mathematics and computer science in which linear programming (LP) and goal programming (GP) are two workhorses which provide solutions to the user. The concept of LP and GP can be applied in animal farming to formulate the least cost balanced ration. Finding the least cost ration which satisfies the animals' need is important because ration cost is the single greatest variable which determines the profitability of dairy farming. Dairy farmers in the Mandya district of Karnataka have very limited feed resources to fulfill the nutrients requirement in terms of crude protein (CP), total digestible nutrients (TDN), calcium (Ca) and phosphorus (P); therefore, one needs a software program to plan a balanced low budget diet. Linear programming and goal programming approaches, alone or in combination, have proved beneficial for finding solutions to ration formulation and diet-related problems of many animals and poultry. This study is a step forward in that direction to provide least cost diet formulation based on nutrient requirements of cattle and buffalo, which has been calculated according to the specifications of the Indian Council of Agricultural Research (ICAR, 2013) and National Research Council (NRC, 2001). Linear programming models for three types of "dairy cattle with body weight 500 kg each and requirement of 10 litre milk yield with 4% of fat content with seventh, eight, and ninth months of pregnancy" and "non-pregnant dairy buffalo weighing 450 kg and yielding 10 L milk with 6% of fat content" are considered on a dry matter basis. Further, a primitive goal programming model for three categories of dairy cattle and non-pregnant buffalo has been formulated by categorizing the goals into a set of priorities. Goal programming models have been developed because there are two high priority objectives: least cost and the dry matter intake to be achieved (if possible). These linear programming models for dairy cattle are comprehended by generalized reduced gradient (GRG) nonlinear, evolutionary, simplex linear programming (LP) and real coded genetic algorithm (RGA) with and without seeding the random number generation methods. The outcome reveals there was no significance difference ($P > 0.05$) found with various techniques adopted for feed preparation, and RGA can be adopted for feed conceptualization. The linear and goal programming model for non-pregnant dairy buffalo was solved using hybrid real coded genetic algorithm, and the results are compared with (RGA), considering different versions like RGA without crossover, RGA without mutation and RGA with crossover and mutation. Here it is observed, however, that RGA without crossover and RGA without mutation operator provide a near to optimal answer, but solutions seem to get stuck in local minima. Hence, RGA with hybrid function provides the optimal solution, and this method can be utilized for cheap feed formulation for dairy cows and buffaloes. This study reveals that the rations of dairy animals can be optimized using real coded genetic algorithm by solving linear and goal programming models of feed formulation.

Acknowledgments

Shrii Saraswatii Namahstubhyam Varade Kaama Ruupini Twaam Aham Praarthane Devii Vidyaadaanam Cha Dehi Me

"I bow to Goddess Saraswati, who fulfils the wishes of the devotees. I pray to her to enlighten me with knowledge. Saraswati is the provider of boons and the one who grants all our desires. She is capable of removing ignorance and bestowing intelligence. I pray to the Goddess to help me in making this work fruitful and make me successful in all my efforts." I am grateful to Lord Ganesha for giving me patience and strength to overcome difficulties, which helped me crossing my way in the accomplishment of this endeavour.

It is hard to say whether it has been grappling with the topic itself which has been the real learning experience or grappling with how to write papers, give talks, work in a group, stay up until the birds start singing and stay focused. In any case, I am indebted to many people for making the time working on my book an unforgettable experience. It would not have been possible to write this book without the help and support of the kind people around me. I acknowledge many known and unknown hands that have helped me in this process. No words could adequately express my gratitude to them, and I shall ever remain indebted to them all. I express my heart with a profound sense of gratitude to my supervisor Dr. Radha Gupta, Professor and Head, Department of Mathematics, Dayananda Sagar College of Engineering, Bangalore. She has oriented and supported me with promptness and care and has always been patient and encouraging in times of new ideas and difficulties. Her excellent quality in teaching the subject will remain in my mind forever. Her hard work, constant patience and determined mind set an example. This book would not have been possible without her help, constant support and patience. Her invaluable help of constructive comments and suggestions throughout my research work have contributed to the progress of this research. I am very much thankful to Dr. D. Rajendran, Principal Scientist, Animal Nutrition Division, National Institute of Animal Nutrition and Physiology (NIANP), Adugodi, Bangalore, for providing primary data and continuous guidance in this research journey. His enormous research experience as well as subject knowledge is source of inspiration for me which helped me to carry this work to this level. He also helped me in improving my writing skills, finding appropriate journals and in making an Excel-based nutrient bound calculator for calculating nutrient requirements of dairy cattle and buffaloes and result validation. Above all, he made me feel as a friend, which I appreciate from my heart. I am deeply grateful to Dr. Sandeep Shastri, Professor and the Vice Chancellor of Vice Chancellor, Jagran Lake City University, Bhopal, who has made me understand the word research. His innovative and systematic way of teaching research methodology has helped me to carry out the work in an effective way. He has provided the right direction to the entire path of research and enlightened and entertained us with his knowledge, experience and skill in this field. I can't imagine my current position without the support from my mother and sister. A formal statement of acknowledgment will hardly meet the end of justice in the matter of the expression of a deep sense of gratitude to my mother, Smt. Premvati Devi. I express my deep sense of love and gratitude for her great patience at all times, constant encouragement and inspiration. I also express my deep sense of gratitude to Dr. Anita Chaturvedi, Professor, Department of Mathematics, FET Jain (Deemed-to-be) University for her kind support and encouragement at all times. I am also very much thankful to Dr. Kokila Ramesh, Department of Mathematics, FET Jain (Deemed-to-be) University for extending her help in times of need. I also express my deep sense of gratitude to Ms. Priya Chakraborty, Department of English, FET Jain (Deemed-to-be) University for extending her help in correcting grammatical errors in this text book.

Authors

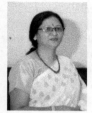

Dr. Radha Gupta earned her M.Sc. degree in mathematics from Agra University, Uttar Pradesh, India, in 1992 and M.Phil. degree in mathematics from the University of Roorkee, Uttarakhand, India, in 1993. She earned her Ph.D. degree in mathematics from Vikram University, Ujjain, Madhya Pradesh, India, in 2011.

From 1993 to 1996, she worked as a research fellow with the Central Building Research Institute, Roorkee, Uttarakhand. From 1999 to 2004, she was a lecturer in SVM PU College Bangalore; from 2004 to 2007 she was a lecturer in the PES Institute of Technology, Bangalore. She moved to the School of Engineering and Technology, Jain University, Bangalore, in 2007 and served the Institution as Associate Professor and Head, Department of Basic Science, till 2015. Since 2015, she has been a professor and department head with the Mathematics Department, Dayananda Sagar College of Engineering, Bangalore. Her research interests include operations research, differential equations, mathematical modelling and statistical analysis.

Dr. Radha Gupta is the author of five books, some conference papers and more than 50 research publications in reputed national and international journals. She is also a reviewer for some prestigious journals. She is a recognized research supervisor from Visvesvaraya Technological University (VTU), Belagavi and a member of many professional bodies. Dr. Radha Gupta was a recipient of the President Gold Medal (from then *President of India, Shri Shankar Dayal Sharma*) for the best student of the year, 1992, Agra University, Uttar Pradesh, and also a recipient of the University Gold Medal for standing first class first in M.Phil. (mathematics) in the year 1993, University of Roorkee, Uttarakhand.

Dr. Ravinder Singh Kuntal is an expert in optimizing and creating user-friendly applications in Microsoft Excel and the Android platform for least cost ration formulation for dairy animals. His research interests include operations research, data analytics, mathematical modelling and statistical analysis. He has worked on these models after eight years of experience in least cost optimization research. He is currently an Assistant Professor of Mathematics in the Faculty of Engineering and Technology, Jain (Deemed-to-be University) Bangalore. He has a total of 11 years of teaching and eight years of research experience. He has published 14 research papers in peer-reviewed journals. He has received many awards for his research work and has bagged the title of Best Paper Award for "Least Cost Formulation for Ruminants" in the International Conference on Applications of Artificial Intelligence and Computational Mathematics (AAICM – 2020). One of his publications also received an acknowledgment of Best Paper Award on "Study of Real Coded Hybrid Genetic Algorithm (RGA) to Find Least Cost Ration for Non-Pregnant Dairy Buffaloes" at the 7th International conference on Soft Computing for Problem Solving (SocPros–2017) December 23–24, 2017, at IIT Bhubaneswar, the Best Paper Award titled "heuristic approach to nonlinear optimization technique" at Research Retreat: Exploring Pathways, Unlocking Ideas" at Jain University. He was named the Best Mathematics Professor of the year in recognition of continuous excellence in teaching, awarded at International Education Awards conference 2020. He has a research collaboration with the NIANP (National Institute of Animal Nutrition and Physiology) Bangalore, India. He also completed consultancy projects for ICAR-NIANP institutions and "Design and Development Least Cost Feed Formulation (LCFF) Application for Goat, Sheep & Camel Using Excel VBA", for King Saud University, Riyadh, Saudi Arabia.

Dr. Vishal Patil is an expert in developing and designing least cost linear programming (LP) and stochastic models and creating user-friendly application in Microsoft Excel and the Android platform. He has built these models after ten years of experience in teaching and research. He has completed consultancy projects for ICAR-NIANP institutions and "Design and Development Least Cost Feed Formulation (LCFF) Application for Goat, Sheep & Camel Using Excel VBA", for King Saud University, Riyadh, Saudi Arabia. He has published ten peer-reviewed international papers. He is an Assistant Professor of Mathematics in the Faculty of Engineering & Technology, Jain (Deemed-to-be University), Bangalore. His major contribution includes research collaboration with NIANP (National Institute of Animal Nutrition and Physiology) Bangalore, India.

Professor D. Rajendran, Principal Scientist, ICAR-National Institute of Animal Nutrition and Physiology, completed his Bachelor of Veterinary Science at Tamilnadu Veterinary and Animal Sciences University, Chennai, in 1997 and his Master in Animal Nutrition at the Indian Veterinary Research Institute, Bareilly. He was a recipient of the Junior Research Fellowship Award during his master's degree. In 2000 he joined West Bengal University of Animal and Fishery Science as a lecturer. He pursued his doctoral degree programme at Madras Veterinary College, Chennai. Professor Rajendran received three Gold Medals during his PhD program, namely the TANUVAS Gold Medal, Dr. Richard Masilamani Memorial Award and TANUVAS Alumni Award. He joined as Assistant Professor in Animal Nutrition at the Veterinary College and Research Institute, Namakkal, Taminadu and established the Feed Mill under a revolving fund project. He conducted research on nano minerals and guided two undergraduate students to receive the ALLTECH Young Scientist Award 2010 and 2011. He joined as senior scientist in 2010 at the ICAR-National Institute of Animal Nutrition and Physiology, Bangalore. His pioneering work on nano technology in animal nutrition for the improvement of bioavailability of mineral is an eye-opener for the application of nano mineral science in animal nutrition. The work was recognized and received best thesis award by the *Animal Nutrition Journal* by Elsevier Pvt. Ltd.

He has 185 publications, including 51 research articles, 12 book chapters, 37 technical articles and 20 teaching manuals. He received seven awards in conferences and seminars of national and international repute. He was invited as guest lecturer by CG Group at Boun Me Thout, DakLak, Vietnam. He successfully guided 12 master degree and five doctoral degree students in the capacity of chairman/member of the advisory committee. He developed four software and two Android apps and published them for public use. He has published five ready reckoners and one diagnostic kit. More than 25000 copies of the ready reckoner were sold and created a revolution in the field of animal nutrition. He has successfully completed 11 externally/institute funded research projects, and currently has five projects in progress. The International Society of Biotechnology conferred the Fellow of International Society of Biotechnology (FISBT) on him in recognition of his contribution and achievements.

Abbreviations

b	Bran Max
BGA	Binary Coded Genetic Algorithm
Ca	Calcium
c/h	Legume/Non-Legume Green
Ck	Cake Max
CP	Crude Protein
d/g	Dry/Green Roughage
DM	Dry Matter
DMI	Dry Matter Intake
EA	Evolutionary Algorithm
GA	Genetic Algorithm
gm/kg	Gram per Kilogram
GP/GPP	Goal Programming/Goal Programming Problem
GRG	Generalized Reduced Gradient
ICAR	Indian Council of Agricultural Research
INR	Indian Rupees
KT	Kuhn-Tucker
lc	Least Cost
LP/LPP	Linear Programming/Linear Programming Problem
NIANP	National Institute of Animal Nutrition and Physiology
NLP/NLPP	Nonlinear Programming/ Nonlinear Programming Problem
NRC	National Research Council
P	Phosphorus
r/c	Roughage/Concentrate
RGA	Real Coded Genetic Algorithm
RHGA	Real Coded Hybrid Genetic Algorithm
RNG	Random Number Generation
RST	Controlled Random Search Technique
SQP	Sequential Quadratic Programming
t	Total (in Kg)
TDN	Total Digestible Nutrients
TMR	Total Mixed Ration

1

Introduction to Animal Nutrition

CONTENTS

1.1 Operational Research

Operational research is a subject field that comprehends a wide range of applications in logical methods to make effective decision-making. Further, operational or operations research emerged while providing the solution to plan efficient military operations during World War II. Operational research is used not only in military operations but also in industry, government, agriculture and animal production. Today's operations research has overlap with many disciplines such as industrial engineering, dairy etc., with the motto of maximizing the profit, performance or yield as well as minimizing the loss, risk or cost of some real-world problems. We cannot give any standard definition to operations research, as its boundaries are not fixed, but as per the Institute for Operations Research and the Management Sciences (INFORMS):

> Operations Research and the Management Sciences are the professional disciplines that deal with the application of information technology for informed decision-making.

Yet this explicit definition is not sufficient, as it is different from a related field. However, operations research is a subfield of applied mathematics. We are using techniques from mathematics such as mathematical modeling, statistical analysis and mathematical optimization to arrive at optimal or near-optimal solutions to complex problems. Therefore, instead of following the INFORMS definition, we use operations research with the help of mathematical optimization to specify

DOI: 10.1201/9781003231714-1

1

techniques and solutions for specific real-time problems. This method includes linear programming, nonlinear programming, integer programming, optimization, the Markov process, queuing theory, goal programming and heuristic algorithms. These techniques would be accepted because they give optimal solutions for specific problems except for the fact that in linear programming, if the problem is not defined in linear equations (equalities or inequalities) or continuous domain, then we cannot apply linear programming algorithms. There are many techniques in operations research which have proven to be very useful in practice. For many real-world optimization problems, operations research provides the method of choice, in particular for those problems that are complex in nature.

1.2 Animal Nutrition

India has the largest livestock population in the world. Livestock is one of the most important economic activities as it plays an important role in growth of Indian agriculture, the growth of Indian economy (it contributes about 4% of national gross domestic product – GDP – and 25% on agricultural GDP) and in livelihood, especially in the rural areas of the country, providing income for most of the family. In dairy farming, feeding cost accounts for about 70% of total operation cost. As per the Government of India Ministry of Agriculture Department of Animal Husbandry, Dairying, and Fisheries, Krishi Bhavan, in the 19th livestock census-2012 all India report, the total milch animals population (cows and buffaloes) has increased to 118.59 million (2012), an increase of 6.75%. The female buffalo population has increased by 7.99% over the previous census, and the total number of female buffaloes was 92.5 million in 2012. The buffalo population increased from 105.3 million to 108.7 million, showing a growth of 3.19%. The population of cows increased by 6.52%, and the total number of cows estimated in 2012 was 122.9 million. As per the Basic Husbandry & Fisheries statistics 2017, the per capita availability of average milk in Karnataka was 291 grams per day during 2016–17, which is less than the 12 top milk-producing states in India, such as Uttar Pradesh. Karnataka has only a 4% share in milk production in year 2016–17. From 2012 to 2016, the cattle population increased from 1.14 million to 1.37 million, with estimated milk production of 5718.22 to 6562.15 (in thousands) in which the average yield per in-milk animal of nondescript/indigenous cows during 2012–13 to 2016–17 in Karnataka was 2.32–2.43 kg/day. Area under fodder crops is increased from 35000 hectares in 2006–07 to 36000 hectares, and permanent pastures and other grazing lands decreased from 930000 hectares to 906000 hectares from 2006–07 to 2013–14 (Basic Animal Husbandry & Fisheries Statistics, 2017). According to Basic Animal Husbandry & Fisheries Statistics 2017 there was a decrease of the cattle population (190 million vs. 199 million) but an increase in buffalo (108 million vs. 105 million) population from the previous census (2012 vs. 2007). These animals contribute about 165.4 million tons of milk production annually (2016–17), in which the major contribution was from buffalo, greater than 49%. Per capita availability of milk in 2010–11 increased from 281 g/d to 355 g/d in 2016–17. In addition, during 2016–17, the share of milk production from cross-breed cows, indigenous cows, nondescript cows and buffaloes was 25.4%, 11.3%, 9.5% and 49.2%, respectively, of total milk production. The increase in population of exotic/ cross-breed cattle and indigenous cattle was 34.8 % and 0.17%, respectively, whereas the population of milk animals (cows and buffaloes) has increased from 77.04 million to 80.52 million. Increasing the productivity of animals is one of the major issues in our country, which can be overcome by developing proper feeding systems to provide balanced nutrients to fulfill their requirements. By looking at increasing demands of animal products such as milk and dairy products, we can see a growth in a new entrepreneurship area with a commercial outlook for which scientific management and sustainability are important components. Nutrients are very important to dairy animals to maintain their body conditions, for milk production with an adequate amount of fat percentage and for maintaining pregnancy at third trimester. These nutrients are provided through feed, and the nutrient requirements are measured in terms of energy, protein, minerals and vitamins. In many developed countries, the standard feeding practice has come through various continuous experiments, evaluation and refinement for decades. But in India, the first published document on scientific feeding for Indian cattle appeared in ICAR bulletin No 25, titled "Nutritive Values of Indian Cattle Feeds and the Feeding of Animals" by Sen (1957). This was later modified by Sen and Ray (1964), and these feeding practices was revised by Sen, Ray and Ranjhan (1978) with some research on Indian breeds. Kearl in 1982 compiled data on nutritional requirements of different livestock species and values of different feedstuffs from various developing countries in a systematic manner. After reviewing these facts, India compiled these standards, and as a result, nutritional requirements of cattle and buffalo were published by ICAR in 1985 and 1998. After this publication, a change in productivity of Indian livestock and nutritive values were experienced in new verity of crop, and modern agriculture practices were introduced, which allows new methodologies for animal nutrition. In 2013, ICAR came out with nutrient requirement of cattle and buffaloes and other species to enhance their productivity. Unfortunately, feeding standards have not been popularized to all dairy farmers due to lack of awareness among farmers as well as lack of resources. In fact, there is a need to provide knowledge of feeding practice to farmers; though there are many government bodies working on these issues in rural areas, there is still need to enhance the overall productivity. Therefore, in present research, an effort has been made by to provide a least cost balanced ration to livestock at different conditions.

1.3 Essential Nutrients

Water is one of the most important nutrients for life. For cattle and buffalo an adequate amount of water is necessary according to body weight, but in general cattle and buffalo need 5.5 to 8.0 and 6.5 to 10.0 litres of water for every 100 kg of body weight per day depending on atmospheric temperature, respectively (Ranjhan, 1998). Water intake may vary according to temperature and dryness of feed; for example if cattle eat healthy grass in spring, they will drink less water than the cattle grazing in summer. Feed contains various amounts of moistures; hence, nutrient contents are expressed in a dry matter (DM) basis to maintain uniformity. For feeding of dairy cattle and buffalo, dry matter is what needs to be considered for feeding other nutrients in adequate quantity and to satisfy animal satiety. Underfeeding as well as overfeeding animals needs to be avoided, as underfeeding causes less production and may lead to nutritional disorder, whereas overfeeding can cause high cost and reproduction issues and excess nutrient excretion, which cause environmental pollution. DM intake (DMI) depends upon body weight of cattle and buffalo, where body weight can be predicted through body measurement (ICAR-NIANP, 2013). Several factors affect DMI including body weight, milk yield, milk fat percentage, environment temperature, density of nutrient in feed, water intake and overall health status, etc., whereas low DMI may lead to nutritional stress and cause less production, infertility and health deterioration.

1.3.1 Energy

Per se, energy is not a nutrient, but it is an important component for all types of body functions which needs to be supplied through diets because dairy cattle and buffalos need to maintain their energy level for body maintenance, reproduction, lactation and growth and during pregnancy. Energy requirement for dairy animal are expressed as total digestible nutrients (TDN), where the requirement of TDN will differ according to animal physiological condition.

1.3.2 Protein

Protein is basically made up of amino acids by peptide bonds, which are used to make tissues. Protein is important for growth and milk production and to maintain body conditions. Livestock use amino acids from digested protein to repair and to build tissues and also utilize microbial protein produced in rumen during the protein degradation process. Because of rumen microbes in cattle, rumen can break down about 80% of protein in the feed and form microbial protein. Protein requirements for dairy animals usually are expressed as crude protein (CP).

1.3.3 Minerals

Minerals are important for various body functions of dairy animals. Minerals, along with proteins, form bone and teeth, and some minerals help in nerve impulse transmission and to carry oxygen. These are basically two types – macro and micro. For dairy animals, the major minerals are macro minerals such as calcium, phosphorus, magnesium, sodium, potassium, chloride and sulphur which is required in diet at a higher level, which is measured as a percentage of dry matter. Based on different physiological conditions of livestock, minerals must be included for optimum performance and health. Therefore, by considering these facts, the required value of DMI, TDN and CP for dairy animals has been calculated as per the ICAR 2013 standards, while values of calcium and phosphorus are calculated according to National Research Council (NRC) 2001 standards. These values are fixed by ICAR and NRC, but a small amount of variation has been incorporated after discussion with qualified animal nutritionists from ICAR-National Institute of Animal Nutrition and Physiology (NIANP), in Adugodi, Bangalore.

1.4 Classification of Feedstuffs

Feed is classified as concentrates and roughage (dry and green) for dairy animals. Common green roughages are cereal grasses, which may be annual or perennial grasses. There are two types of green roughage, cereals and leguminous. Legumes have advantage over cereal grass due to their nitrogen fixing, which means that these plants contain more protein than cereal grass because they can fix atmospheric nitrogen (with the help of bacteria), and they are not dependent on nitrogen content present in the soil. Dry roughages include straw from rice, barley wheat and ragi, and stovers from sorghum, maize, Bajra etc., are widely used as dry roughage in feed. Roughage is feed which have high fiber content, usually more than 18% on DM basis. The concentrate contains high amount of nutrients with less fiber usually less than 18% on DM basis. The most common concentrate is cereal grains such as maize grain, sorghum grain, broken rice, wheat etc., as well as oil seed cake of various kinds and milling by-products. These concentrates are very rich in energy compared to roughage. Concentrates have a high amount of energy (TDN) and less fiber (less than 18% of DM); hence it is denser than roughages. Nutrient requirement of a dairy cow/ buffalo is calculated based on the nutrient requirement prescribed by ICAR-NIANP (2013). These requirements include DM (kg/d), TDN (kg/d), CP (g/d), Ca (g/d) and P (g/d). The nutrient requirements of a cow/buffalo are met by feeding the required proportion of concentrate and green and dry roughages. This required proportion needs to be calculated, and the final ration (amount of feed eaten by cow for a day) is prepared by mixing green and dry roughages and concentrate together. The mixture of concentrate and green and dry fodder is called the total mixed ration. While preparing feed, all the nutrients (DM (kg/d), TDN (kg/d), CP (g/d), Ca (g/d) and P (g/d)) must be balanced, and at the same time cost of the final feed should be minimized. Preparation of least cost feed formulation is a challenging task for any nutritionist, and application of optimization techniques of operational research will provide solutions for this kind of problem. A goal-seeking program of operational research will be a useful tool to formulate rations for dairy animals. In this program, required nutrients (DM (Kg/d), TDN (Kg/d), CP (g/d), Ca (g/d) and P (g/d)) of a dairy for physiological state (yielding 10 litre/d milk production with 4% fat and pregnancy in third trimester) are fixed as constraints, and the amount of feed required in terms of concentrate and green and dry fodder is calculated by applying heuristic techniques (genetic algorithm). Some of the common feedstuffs commonly used for ration formulation with its nutrient values are listed in Table 1.1. While formulating least cost balanced ration, the selection of feedstuffs is depending upon the availability in the respective region.

TABLE 1.1

Nutrient Content of Common Feeds and Fodder for Dairy Cattle and Buffalo on DM Basis

Name of the ingredients	DM %	CP %	TDN %	Ca %	P %
Green roughage					
Bajra Napier CO-4 grass	25	8	52	0.144	0.09
Maize fodder	25	8	60	0.53	0.14
Sorghum Co-FS 29 fodder	90	7	50	0.12	0.09
Berseem	90	5	45	0.65	0.05
Dry roughage					
Paddy straw	90	5.13	40	0.18	0.08
Maize stover	90	3	42	0.145	0.027
Ragi straw	90	6	42	0.15	0.09
Concentrate					
Maize	90	8.1	79.2	0.018	0.27
Soya DOC	90	42	70	0.018	0.225
Copra DOC	90	22	70	0.036	0.9
Cotton DOC	90	32	70	0.036	0.9
Wheat bran	75	12	70	1.067	0.093
Gram chunnies	90	17	60	0.108	0.234
Cotton seed	90	16	110	0.3	0.62
Chickpea husk	90	18	45	0.3	0.62
Concentrate mix Type I	90	22	70	0.5	0.45
Concentrate mix Type II	90	20	65	0.5	0.4
Minerals					
Calcite	97	0	0	36	0
Grit	96	0	0	36	0
MM	90	0	0	32	6
DCP	90	0	0	24	16
Soda bicarbonate	90	0	0	0	0
Salt	90	0	0	0	0
TM mix	98	0	0	0	0
Urea	95	287.5	0	0	0

1.5 Application Area

According to past surveys, it was clear that farmers are not feeding dairy cattle according to the nutrient requirement suggested by the scientific community due to unawareness and unavailability of proper feedstuffs. Animal feed plays a large role in the sustainability performance of animal production systems, and the choice of diet affects animal production. Diet formulation could be a method of blending totally different feedstuffs in appropriate proportions so that animals can consume it, and it provides required nutrients to cattle.

In India many livestock organizations have reported shortages of feedstuff; therefore, Karnataka dairy farmers faced many problems in increasing the performance of livestock due to the inadequacy of feedstuff in both quality and quantity. In addition to that, many feed resources that could have a major impact on livestock production are either unused or poorly utilized by the farmers, and a critical factor in this regard is lack of awareness about feedstuffs available in their respective regions and nutritional values. Even though in the past many decades a reasonable growth has been seen in dairy animals, it is necessary to increase their productivity (Ravinder, 2017). Milk production is one of the major contributors to the growth of the Indian economy, so it is necessary to formulate a low-cost, balanced ration for livestock. To formulate the ration, it is necessary to have the best possible information about feedstuffs, nutrients contained inside the feedstuffs and, additionally, which sort of dairy animal should be supplied with such a ration to guarantee an ideal production at a cheaper rate. Various categories of dairy cows and buffaloes have diverse prerequisites for vitality (sugars and fats), proteins, minerals and vitamins to keep up their various functions, such as body repair, proliferation, milk production and fetus growth during the third trimester of pregnancy. The formulated ration should be rich in energy, protein, phosphorus, minerals and vitamins; in addition, it ought not create any genuine stomach-related problems or unfavorable impacts on the dairy cattle (Gupta et al., 2013a). For example, pregnant cattle at third trimester not only require nutrition for body maintenance but also for milk production with adequate amount of fat percentage and fetus growth. It also is necessary to avoid the overfeeding of nutrients to cattle (Mudgal et al., 2003), which may affect milk production and their health. For this reason, an animal nutrition expert is required for information about nutrition requirements.

2

Review of Literature

CONTENTS

2.1 Introduction

Feed formulation is the process of quantifying the amounts of different feed ingredients that need to be put together to form a single uniform mixture (diet) for animals that supplies all their nutrient requirements. It is concerned with the allocation of nutrient ingredients to the animal in terms of yield and weight gain at the least possible cost. It is one of the central operations of the animal industry, as the performance and the optimal growth of animals is entirely dependent on their feed intake. To meet the animals' requirement at a particular stage of production, it is very important to formulate the diet efficiently with low cost, as feed costs account for 40–80% of the total costs in animal production (Pond et al., 1995), 75–85% in pig production (Gallenti, 1997: 15–19) and over 60% in poultry production (Rose, 1997), and in milk production feed costs are the largest expense (Bath, 1985: 1579–1584). Therefore, procedures that reduce feed costs are likely to increase net incomes in agriculture. Feed formulation is one of the areas that one can use to reduce the cost of feed (Nabasirye et al., 2011: 221–226). Rations for livestock should be formulated in such a way that they should supply all essential nutrients and energy to maintain the vital physiological functions of growth, reproduction and health of animals. To formulate the low-cost diet, planning the linear programming-based diet formulation has come into existence with the help of mathematicians. This method is widely used in commercial dairy farms and commercially available software. The least cost formulation of rations based on linear programming optimizes the combination of feed ingredients which supplies the required amount of nutrients at least cost (Rossi, 2004). The major nutrients to

DOI: 10.1201/9781003231714-2

be supplied in a diet are energy, protein and minerals such as calcium and phosphorus for maintenance, growth, pregnancy and milk production of dairy animals. These nutrients should be supplied in required quantity to meet the specific performance targets. These entire concepts need a professional knowledge of animal nutrition to consider the requirements of the nutrients and animals' capability to digest and then assimilate the nutrients from various available ingredients.

Livestock ration formulation models are developed for commercial purposes as well as for development, using various mathematical techniques for several decades. Some of them use the Pearson's square method: the Pearson's square ration formulation procedure is designed for simple rations and has been used for many years. It is direct and easy to follow and is useful in balancing protein requirements. The limitation of this technique is that it satisfies only one nutrient requirement and uses only two feed ingredients. It therefore has limited application where farmers must formulate diets balanced for protein, energy, minerals and least cost (Chakeredza et al., 2008: 2925–2933). The simultaneous equation method is one more method that uses a simple algebraic equation. The advantage of this over the Pearson's square method is that it is useful in considering more than two feed ingredients at a time when balancing rations is more complex. The two by two matrix method solves two nutrient requirements using two feed ingredients. A 2×2 matrix is set and a series of equations are done to come up with the solution to the problem.

Trial and error method: This method is used for formulating rations for swine and poultry. As the name implies, the formulation is manipulated until the nutrient requirements of the animal are reached. This method makes possible a diet formulation that meets all the requirements of the animal. The major limitation of this method is that it is laborious and time consuming before one approaches a better solution. Many mathematical programming techniques are being used to formulate rations, such as linear programming, multiple-objective programming, goal programming, separable programming, quadratic programming, nonlinear programming and genetic algorithm. In the present work, we are discussing linear and nonlinear programming techniques in animal diet formulation.

2.2 Linear Programming in Ration Formulation

The history of linear programming (LP) goes back to 1947, when George Dantzig and his team were working in the U.S. Air Force and found that many military programming and planning problems can be formulated to minimize/maximize a linear form of profit/cost function whose variables were restricted to values satisfying a system of linear constraints. Linear programming has its application in various decision-making processes such as human diet, portfolio optimization, transportation problems, crew scheduling airlines etc. In many algorithms for optimization problems, linear programming is used to solve a sub-problem where, if the feasible region is a subset of the non-negative portion defined by linear equations or inequalities, and the objective function to be minimized or maximized is linear, then we have a linear programming problem or LPP (Meyer, 1985). Selecting the best alternative out of many possibilities is called optimization. Patrick and Schaible (1980: 417–458) stated that LP is technically a mathematical procedure for obtaining a value weighting solution to a set of simultaneous equations. The earliest systematic method for numerically solving an LPP was developed by Dantzig and is called the simplex method. The simplex method is an algebraic iterative procedure which exactly solves an LPP problem in a finite number of steps or gives an indication that there is no solution or an unbounded solution. Most of the computational techniques currently in use are based on the simplex approach. Most companies would like to maximize profits or minimize costs with limited resources; such issues can be characterized as LPP. There are hundreds of applications of linear programming in agriculture (Taha, 1987). One of the major applications is in livestock feed formulation. Linear programming is the common method of least cost feed formulation, and for the last 50 years it has been used as an efficient technique in ration formulation. It has formed the basis for livestock feed formulation since Waugh (1951) defined the feeding problem in a mathematical form. He was not an animal nutritionist by profession but, as he confessed, was trying to look for something suitable to lighten the animal nutritionist's job. Since then, LP has been used widely for diet formulation. While formulating rations by linear programming, first and foremost, all available raw materials and feed ingredients are selected which are to be included in ration, and then a set of constraints on feed ingredients is set up. An objective function is then formulated as per the available feed ingredients and constraints to achieve the objective. While constructing a linear programming model, the following assumptions are made:

Linearity: Feed formulation by LP is mainly based on the linearity between animal yield and nutrient ingredients included in the diet. Linearity means the amount of each resource used and its contribution to the objective function is proportional to the value of each decision variable.

Simple objective: There is single objective (can be either maximization of animal yield or minimization of cost of the diet) which is a mathematical function.

Additivity: This means that the sum of resources used by different activities must be equal to the total quantity of resources used by each activity for all the resources (Dantzig, 1963).

Certainty: While formulating a linear model for animal rations, it is assumed that all parameters of the model and consumption of resources are known with certainty.

Divisibility: It is assumed that all inputs into the ration are infinitely divisible. Perfect divisibility of outputs and resources must exist.

Non-negativity: Decision variables cannot be added to the final objective function in a negative way. More precisely, the solution values of decision variables are allowed to assume continuous and non-negative values.

Finiteness: The constraints and the variables must be finite so that the ration can be programmed. Hence, a finite number of activities and constraints must be employed (Gale et al., 1951).

Proportionality: This implies that the contribution of each variable to the objective function is directly proportional to each variable (Al-Deseit, 2009).

All these assumptions indicate that the objective function and all the constraints must be characterized by a linear relationship among decision variables in the LP model. LP has been used as a basic tool for animal feed formulation since 1950. Interest in livestock ration formulation accelerated, and a laboratory diet was considered as an important variable. During the 1970s, the American Institute of Nutrition, National Academy of Science, Institute of Laboratory Science, Institute of Laboratory Animal Resources and Laboratory Animal Centre Diets Advisory Committee supported the use of standard reference diets in biomedical research. A linear model was developed (Van de Panne and Popp, 1963) to formulate an optimized composition of cattle feed. In this LP model, the coefficients of constraints can be considered as stochastic. Feed utilization is described in terms of feed ration, response gain, biological function and economic efficiency. Nutritional, genetic and physiological responses are interpreted as a function of gain and feed intake (Meyer and Garrett, 1967); the incorporation of information on animal performance into the linear programming derivation of optimum livestock rations is taken into consideration (Townsley, 1968). Another model was developed using linear approximation of chance constrained programming (Olson and Swenseth, 1987). The LP model can be solved for a complicated set of nutrient requirements to give a relatively well-balanced ration (Haar and Black, 1991: 541–556). Sklan and Dariel (1993) developed a nutritional program for high producing dairy herds to attain efficient and profitable levels of milk production. The main goal in the application of LP in feed formulation is the production of least cost rations that produce satisfactory results. A nutrition program was developed for high producing dairy herds to attain efficient and profitable satisfactory results. It has been widely used in livestock rations (Lara, 1993: 321–334), and to formulate feeds, nutritionists should be knowledgeable in diet specifications as well as result interpretations. LP is one of the most important techniques to allocate the available feedstuffs in a least cost broiler ration formulation (Dantzig, 1951; Aletor, 1986; Ali and Leeson, 1995). Olorunfemi et al. (2001) reviewed extensively the use of linear programming in the least cost formulation for aquaculture. Olorunfemi et al. (2001) also applied linear programming into duckweed utilization in low-cost feed formulation for broiler starter. In 2002, Darmon used LP as a tool to optimize human nutrition. A model developed by Tedeschi et al. (2004) is used to represent the efficiency of nutrient use in relation to profitability of dairy farms. Guevara in 2004 developed a cost analysis spreadsheet and validated the efficacy on milking and custom heifer operations. A stochastic linear programming-based Excel workbook was developed that consists of two worksheets illustrating linear and stochastic program methods. This Excel sheet was set up to calculate the margin of safety value according to probability. The multiple-objective programming was applied for feed formulation with the objective of minimizing the nutrient and minimizing cost. This study introduced a dual model in linear programming to obtain the price of resources that take part in optimization. The price of nutrients resource showed degree of influence of a diet's cost by increasing or decreasing the expected nutrient values. When the price of some kind of resource is zero, it means that reaching this nutrient value does not have influence on a special diet least cost within a particular value (Xiong et al., 2003). Therefore, for the past seven decades, use of linear programming technique has been used to formulate least cost dairy feed (Waugh, 1951; Rehman and Romero, 1987; Zhang and Roush, 2002; Hadrich et al., 2008; Zgajnar and Kavcic, 2008; Al-Deseit, 2009; Almasad et al., 2011; Saxena, 2011a).

2.2.1 Linear Programming Based Software

A few software packages are available based on linear programming for feed formulation such as FEEDLIVE, FEEDMU, WINFEED, ECOMIX, BESTMIX, OPTIMIX, MIXIT, WINPAS, EGGOPRO, FEEDMANIA etc. FEEDLIVE software is meant for feed formulation, and it is bilingual for Thai and English. FEEDMU is simple feed formulation software which is based on the trial and error method and simplex method of linear programming. FEEDMU is upgraded; the new version is FEEDMU2, which uses .NET framework 2.0 technology. FEED FORMULATION is software used to formulate an optimum diet. WINFEED is a very simple and straightforward software which prepares least cost formula diets for ruminants and non-ruminants by using linear and stochastic programming. LINDO (Linear Interactive and Discrete Optimizer), MATLAB, GAMS (General Algebraic Modeling System) and Microsoft Excel Solver are some of the numerous packages dedicated to solving LP problems (Nabasirye, 2011). There are many advantages of using a computer for feed formulation. Some of them are:

- It is convenient and saves manpower.
- It eliminates human error both in calculation and in speed.
- It allows least cost ration formulation using specific information fed into the computer.
- It is a choice for commercial feed millers who handle a large number of ingredients.
- Least cost minimizes the cost of rations given a certain set of ingredients and their nutritional content, which is done in real time using a computer.

(Afolayan, 2008: 1596–1602)

2.2.2 Limitations of Linear Programming in Ration Formulation

However, there are many limitations in using linear programming (LP) while formulating rations, which lies in exclusive reliance of cost. It is very rigid assumption, as more often the decision maker is not interested in an economically optimal ration that achieves a compromise amongst several conflicting objectives such as minimization of cost, imbalance of nutrients supplies and satisfaction of conditions such as the calcium–phosphorus ratio, roughage–concentrate ratio etc. Another weakness of LP is the rigidity with which given nutritional requirements must be met (Rehman and Romero, 1984). Briefly, linear programming is an effective tool of finding the least possible cost of a diet that satisfies a set of nutrient specifications. Although LP has been used widely in practice, with noticeable success (Black and Hlubik, 1980), the assumptions considered while formulating the linear model remain its weakness. Linear programming optimal solutions are based on a linearity assumption which in practice may not be true. Since varying constraints need to be considered, the feed mixing problem has become increasingly difficult to solve using linear programming alone. In varying situations, LP is found insufficient to overcome all the complexities of the problem. It suffers unnecessarily from over-rigid specification of nutritional and other requirements. Some relaxation of the constraints imposed would not seriously effect an animal's well-being and performance.

Over the years, several issues have arisen in feed mixing problems such as ingredient variability. Among them are that the nutrient levels of feed ingredients are unstable and fluctuate (Munford, 1996; Panne and Popp, 1963), that there can be a nutrient imbalance in the final solution and that price variability means prices of feed ingredients are not constant, making the solution infeasible. These problems include the singularity of the objective function and the rigidity of the constraint set. The singularity of the objective function refers to the reliance on cost alone as the most important factor in determining the composition of the ration. Lara (1993) also criticizes practical applications of LP due to the restrictions placed on decision makers' preferences through a singular objective function. Producers are likely to have many objectives in mind while formulating a ration (Tozer and Stokes, 2001). Mitani and Nakayama (1997: 131–139) pointed out three limitations of linear programming model while formulating the ration:

> LP models assume nutrients levels are fixed; however, nutrient levels in feed ingredients are unstable and fluctuating. When the variability among ingredients is neglected, the probability of meeting nutrient restriction is only 50% (Pesti and Siela, 1999). It is hard to determine a good balance of nutrients in the final solution of the linear programming method. If only the minimum levels of nutrient requirements are placed, there is a probability for nutrient imbalance to arise in the final solution. When the variation is small, the quality of balanced nutrients improves. (Zhang and Roush, 2002). The constraint is over-rigidity of nutritional specification and requirement, which means no constraint violation is allowed in LP. This normally leads to an infeasible solution.

2.2.3 Overcoming the Limitations of Linear Programming

Keeping the limitation of LP in mind, various techniques have been proposed in the field of ration formulation such as goal programming, multi-objective goal programming, multi-objective fractional programming, nonlinear programming, chance constrained programming, quadratic programming and risk formulation. All these methods have advantages. However, goal programming and the integrated linear goal programming approach and its application in the ration formulation problem will be discussed at length in Chapters 4, 5 and 6.

2.3 Nonlinear Programming

In linear programming models, the characteristic assumption is the linearity of the objective and constraint functions. Although this assumption holds in many practical situations, we still come across many situations where the objective function and/or some or all of the constraints are nonlinear functions. Such problems are referred as nonlinear programming problems (NLPP). If the objective function and the constraints are all convex functions (a function which, when plotted, results in a curve always curving upwards or not curving at all is called a convex function), the problem is said to be a convex programming problem. The method of solving an LP problem is based on the property that the optimal solution lies at one or more extreme points of the feasible region. This limits our search to corner points, and a finite solution is obtained after a finite number of iterations, as in the simplex method. But this is not true for an NLPP. In such problems, the optimal solution can be located at any point along the boundaries of the feasible region or even within the region. And due to nonlinearity of the objective function and constraints, it becomes difficult to differentiate between the local and global solution. Every linear programming problem can be solved by the simplex method, but there is no single technique which can be claimed to efficiently solve each and every nonlinear optimization problem. In fact, a technique which is efficient for one nonlinear optimization problem may be highly inefficient for solving another NLPP. A variety of computational techniques for solving NLPP are available (Himmelblau, 1972; McCormick, 1970). However, an efficient method for the solution of a general NLPP is still a subject of research. There is a wide variety of nonlinear programming problems. Some of the most important types are constrained and unconstrained NLPP, separable programming, convex programming, non-convex programming, quadratic programming and so on. In a linear-constrained NLPP, all the constraints are of a linear type, and the objective function is nonlinear. And in a nonlinear-constrained NLPP, all the constraints are nonlinear. Many have tried to use unconstrained optimization methods for solving nonlinear problems with constraints. A successful and frequently used approach is to define an auxiliary unconstrained problem such that the solution of the unconstrained problem yields the solution of the constrained problem. Goldfarb has extended the Davidon–Fletcher–Powell method to handle problems with linear constraints utilizing the concept of gradient projection (Goldfarb, 1969: 739–764). The method was generalized by Davies to handle nonlinear constraints (Davies, 1970). Box developed a constrained version of the simplex method (Broyden, 1967: 386–381). Another method that uses the simplex technique in constrained optimization was proposed by Dixon (1973a: 23–32). Another important class of methods used for solving a constrained NLPP is known as penalty function methods. In these methods the constrained problem is converted into an unconstrained problem or a sequence of unconstrained problems in which there is a severe penalty for the violation of the constraints. Another class of methods for solving an NLPP is the family of exact penalty function methods. The pioneering work in this field has been done by McCormick (1983). The sequential linear programming approach for constrained optimization problems finds the optimal solution by repeated linear approximation of a nonlinear problem and using linear programming techniques to solve it. Attempts have also been made to obtain the solution of both constrained and unconstrained optimization problems by solving the Kuhn–Tucker (KT) conditions directly. Methods under this category are sometimes classified as multiplier methods. Quasi-Newton type methods have been used to obtain the solution to the system of equations representing KT conditions (Powell, 1977). He also tried to obtain solutions to constrained and unconstrained NLPP by using a least square algorithm for solving the system of nonlinear equations representing the KT condition of the problem. In the absence of convexity, the methods discussed here at the most guarantee a local optimal solution. Keeping in view the practical necessity and the availability of fast computing machines, many computational techniques are being developed to find the global optimal solution. The methods for solving global optimization problems are broadly classified as deterministic and probabilistic methods. The deterministic methods try to guarantee that a neighborhood of the global optima is attained. Such methods do not use any stochastic techniques but rely on a thorough search of the feasible domain. They are applicable to a restricted class of functions only, such as Lipschitz continuous functions. In stochastic or probabilistic methods, two phases are generally employed. In the first phase, or the global phase, the function is evaluated at a number of randomly sampled points. In the second phase, also called the local phase, these points are manipulated by local searches to yield a possible candidate for the global minima. These methods are preferred over the deterministic methods because they are applicable to a wider class of functions. Some of the earlier methods of this category are pure random search methods by Bremermann and Anderson (1989) and Brooks (1958: 244–251). Dixon suggested a method in which any local search method can be used to search the global solution by starting repeatedly from different initial points chosen stochastically. Price presented a controlled random search technique (RST) method in which the simplex approach is used on a random sample of points to yield a better point at each iteration and the method in the limit converges to the point of global minima Dixon (1972a, 1972b, 1973a, 1973b, 1976) and Bharti (1994) have updated the RST method of Price for solving the constrained NLPP (Dixon 1973a).

Bharti has tried to improve the performance of various controlled random search algorithms (1994). Linear programming is an effective method of finding the least possible cost of a unit that satisfies a set of nutrient specifications. An animal's nutritional requirements hold constant only within a single performance level. Changes in diet composition may cause variations in feed intake, animal's nutritional requirements and animal performance. The traditional LP formulation ignores animal performance and feed intake. There are multiple least cost diets at different levels of nutrient concentrations and corresponding animal performances. Thus, a single LP formulation will not necessarily converge to the minimum cost of production or maximum profit, both nonlinear functions of diet composition (Tedeschi et al., 2005). Low-cost balanced ration formulation for livestock involves omitting ingredients with an inclusion rate below some fixed threshold and rounding other ingredients to realistic weighing quantities. It is possible to incorporate these constraints, but then it will not be possible to solve by linear programming, as the nonlinear effect of variables will then be included (Saxena, 2011c: 1–5). It is necessary to control a ratio of nutrients in a formulation – for example, a simple ratio such as that of calcium to phosphorus, or a more complicated one such as forage dry matter to concentrated dry matter in a ruminant complete diet. Also controlling the dry matter percentage as-fed in a diet involving wet feeds is ratio constraint. Ratio constraints are nonlinear and fall outside the scope of a linear programming framework (Munford, 2005, 1989).

The primary objective of feed formulation is to generate a formula to meet the specifications set for it at the lowest possible cost. The inherent variability in the nutrient composition of feed ingredients represents a major risk factor in formulation. The risk associated with nutrient variability must be handled diligently by feed manufacturers. While under-delivery of nutrients is detrimental to feed performance, over-formulating, that is, specifying nutrients more than requirements is wasteful and expensive. Nott and Combs (1967) suggested that nutrient variability in the feed formulation process could be managed by a margin of safety for the nutrients. They recommended an adjustment of the nutrient means by subtracting 0.5 of the nutrient standard deviation. However, nutrient adjustments are not appropriate for a linear program. Technically, it is assumed that input values such as nutrient levels, animal requirements and ingredient costs in a linear program are linear and are known with certainty. Because the variances of nutrients are used in the formulation, the algorithm is the square of the standard deviation. Therefore, nutrient variation as a nonlinear input variable violates the assumptions of linearity and certainty for the LP. Any attempt to adjust a linear program for nutrient variability results in costly over-formulation of the ration. The most appropriate feed formulation method is the use of stochastic programming (William et al., 1994). It is a nonlinear approach to feed formulation, and it is a refinement in providing margins of safety for feed formulation. Stochastic refers to the variability of nutrients and the probability of meeting the nutrient requirement. It is therefore a method of feed formulation that can effectively incorporate nutrient variability into the formulation process to meet animal requirements with a measured level of certainty. The LP method is applied as an effective method to achieve the least cost of feed. But most of the time the price of products and the energy density are ignored in formulating diets.

A nonlinear programming optimization model was developed to maximize the margin over feed cost for broiler feed formulation. The model identifies the optimal feed mix that maximizes profit margin. The NLPP method illustrated the effects of changes in different variables on the optimum energy density, performance and profitability and was compared with conventional LP (Guevara, 2004: 147–151). The study done by Guevara suggests that nonlinear programming can be more useful than conventional linear programming to optimize performance response to energy density in broiler feed formulation because an energy level does not need to be set. In this method, optimum metabolizable energy level and performance were found by using Excel Solver NLP. Eila, Lavvaf and Farahvash showed that the optimum level of energy could be obtained by a nonlinear model depending on the income over cost of energy, so that the price of the produced egg mass is considered as well as the cost of energy density to achieve the maximum amount of benefit (Eila et al., 2012: 1302–1306). Chavas, Kliebenstein and Crenshaw used nonlinear programming to find the diets and rates of gain for swine when neither the length of the feeding program nor the market weights were fixed (1985: 636–646). A model of dynamically optimal cattle purchasing, feeding and selling decisions was constructed and a simple static model developed to closely approximate dynamically optimal decisions. The models were solved using nonlinear programming software, MINOS (Hertzler, 1988: 7–17). Iterative linear programming is used to solve two NLPPs of animal diet formulation (Tozer, 2000: 443–451). To overcome the drawback of linear approximation of the objective function for diet formulation, a mathematical model based on the NLP technique was developed by Pratiksha Saxena to measure animal performance in terms of milk yield and weight gain. The result of developed model was compared with the linear model, and the comparison shows that NLP gives better results for maximization of animal yield and weight gain and represents simultaneous effects of all variables together (Saxena, 2011a: 106–108).

2.4 Goal Programming

Goal programming (GP) is like a linear programming model which allows multiple goals to be satisfied at a time. Multiple goals are sometimes given priority according to weights to meet the various goals. It is a branch of multi-objective optimization, which in turn is branch of multi-criteria decision analysis (MCDA), also known as the multi-criteria decision making (MCDM) process. Hence, goal programming is an extension of linear or nonlinear programming involving an objective function with multiple objectives. While developing a goal-programming model, the decision variables of the model are to be defined first. Then the managerial goals related to the problems are to be listed and ranked in order of priority. Since it may be very difficult to rank these goals on a cardinal scale, an ordinal ranking is usually applied to each of the goals. It may not always be possible to fully achieve every goal specified by the decision maker. Thus, goal programming is often referred to as a lexicographic procedure in which the various goals are satisfied in order of their relative importance. The general mathematical model of the goal programming problem (GPP) is as follows:

$$\text{Minimize } (Z) = \Sigma_{i \in m} \, (d_i^+ + d_i^-) \text{ Subjected to} : \sum\nolimits_{j=1}^{n} (a_{ij} x_j + d_i^- - d_i^+) = g_i$$

where, d_i^+, d_i^-, $x_j \geq 0$ and $(i = 1,2 \ldots m)$, $(j = 1,2 \ldots n)$.

Here d_i^+ is the positive deviation variable from overachieving the ith goal; d_i^- is the negative deviation variable from underachieving the ith goal, and x_j is the decision variables; a_{ij} is the decision variable coefficient. In the weights method, the single objective function is the weighted sum of the functions representing the goals of the problem. The weights goal-programming model is of the form:

$$\text{Minimize } (Z) = \Sigma_{i \in m} \, \{di(W_i^+ + W_i^-)\}, \text{ Subjected to} : \sum\nolimits_{j=1}^{n} (a_{ij} x_j + d_i^+ - d_i^-) = g_i,$$

where d_i^+, d_i^-, $x_j \geq 0$ and $(i = 1,2 \ldots m)$, $(j = 1,2 \ldots n)$. Here W_i^+ and W_i^- are nonnegative constraints and can be real numbers representing the relative weights assigned within a priority level to the deviational variables. The parameter d_i^+ represents positive weights that reflect the decision maker's preference regarding the relative importance of each goal, while d_i^- is the negative weights of the decision maker's preference. The determinant of the specific values of these weights is subjective. The objective of goal programming is to minimize the deviation to find the solution for which the deviation is at minimum. Therefore, to overcome the limitation of LP in diet formulation, a multiple criteria decision-making technique was introduced by Romero and Rehman (1984). In 1992 Lara and Romero used the concept of Rehman and Romero (1987) and then applied a multiple goal programming (MGP) model to introduce the relaxation of nutrient constraints. Lara and Romero (1994) extended their work, as the relaxation of constraints could reduce the ration cost. They considered nutritional requirements as targets which might or might not be achieved. This MGP model is solved using a multiple criteria mathematical programming technique known as the interactive method. The use of this interactive method is to perform a search over a set of feasible diets. The work of Mitani and Nakayama (1997) is also an early contribution in diet formulation. Lara (1993) introduced a second objective, maximization of the inclusion in the diet of the ingredients available on the farm in addition to least cost. This work is introduced in a nonlinear framework because the second objective is considered in fractional form. Tozer and Stokes (2001) used multiple objective programming to reduce nutrient excretion from dairy cows through incorporation of a nutrient excretion function into the ration formulation framework. To reduce the nutrient excretion load, rations are formulated to minimize cost and nitrogen and phosphorus excretion using MGP. Jean dit Bailleul et al. (2001) also developed a multiple objective optimization method to minimize the cost and excess nitrogen in pig diets. Zhang and Roush (2002) introduced two objectives minimizing the cost and the nutrient variabilities for protein, methanone and lysine. MGP applies the same concepts as GP but is different in terms of modelling the objective separately. Therefore, GP and MGP have an advantage in handling multiple objectives, including nutrient variability and reducing nutrient imbalance problems. Castrodeaza et al. (2005) formulated pig rations considering economic and environmental objectives, incorporating advanced nutritional concepts in ratio form and by using an interactive method by multiple objective fractional programming. They considered the cost of feed, the lysine/energy ratio, deviation with regard to the ideal values of the percentage content of amino acids in the protein and the amount of phosphorus. Zgajnar and associates (Zgajnar and Kavcic, 2008, 2009; Zgajnar et al., 2009) also combined LP and weighted GP to find the optimal ration cost with balanced nutritional requirement. One of the primary objectives was to overcome the limitation of linear programming such as LP rigidity and not satisfying primary constraints.

2.5 Genetic Algorithm

A genetic algorithm (GA) is a search algorithm which is based on principles inspired by natural genetic populations to evolve solutions to problems (Holland, 1975; Goldberg, 1989). The main concept is to maintain the population of chromosomes, which amounts to candidate solution to a complex problem that evolves over time through a process of competition. Each chromosome in the population has fitness to determine which chromosome should be used to form new chromosomes during the process, which is called selection. The new chromosomes are created using genetic operators such as crossover and mutation [Goldberg (1989), Holland (1975)]. GAs has great history of success in search problems; the reason for this is their ability to exploit the information about an initially unknown search space in order to bias subsequent searches into useful subspaces, that is, their adaptation. This is the key factor, particularly in large, poorly understood search space problems where classical and old conventional techniques are inappropriate in offering a good search space. Although there are many variants of GA, the fundamental mechanism operates on a population of individuals and consists of three operations: a) creating initial population, b) evaluation of individual fitness, c) formation of a gene pool by selection procedure and d) recombining them using crossover and mutation procedures. In 1998, F. Herrera et al., reviewed the features of real-coded genetic algorithms in which different models of genetic operators and some mechanisms available for studying the behavior of this type of GA have been compared. This review stated that initially the use of RCGA appeared in applications such as chemo metric applications (Lucasius and Kateman, 1989) and use of meta operators (Davis, 1989). Real coded GA has been used mainly for numerical optimization in continuous domains. Later, in 1994, Darrell Whitey covered the canonical genetic algorithm as well as more experimental forms of genetic algorithm, including parallel island models and parallel cellular genetic algorithms. He also illustrates genetic searches by hyperplane sampling and reviewed the theoretical foundation of genetic algorithms which include the fundamental theorem of a genetic algorithms called a "schema theorem" (Holland, 1975) as well as an exact model of the canonical genetic algorithm. Therefore, GA has been used for solving nonlinear programming models as well as multi-objective programming models. It focuses on the initialization process, evaluation process, selection process, crossover and mutation for the nonlinear goal programming problem and concluded that GA is effective for nonlinear GPPs (Zheng et al., 1996; Gen and Cheng, 1997; Deb, 1999; Kumar et al., 2012). In 2014 a combined LP with GP for feed formulation displayed the dip in cost as a major advantage of using the goal-programming approach (Ghosh et al., 2014). Therefore, in view of an exhaustive review of literature, it is observed that no techniques are suitable for formulating rations in a least cost manner for dairy cattle; thus, a comparative study was planned to find a suitable technique that is farmer friendly and can be adopted at the farm level.

3

Tools and Techniques

CONTENTS

3.1 Computation of LP Model Using MS-Excel Based Solver

There are mathematical software packages such as Lingo, Mathematica, TORA, MATLAB, and Excel Solver, etc., which are available widely. Excel Solver, Lingo and Mathematica are freely available, whereas one needs to use a licensed version of MATLAB provided by the university. All this software can be used to solve linear and nonlinear programming problems. The MS-Excel-based spreadsheet is more popular and widely used because Excel-based spreadsheets provide an easy environment for data entry as well as data editing. Due to this, one can gain understanding of how to construct linear models. An MS-Excel based tool known as "Solver" is available to formulate and solve ration formulation problems. The importance of this tool was discussed by Macdonald (1995). Solver can be found in the tool menu of an Excel sheet; if this tool is not found in the tool menu, then it can be added by clicking on Add-Ins in the tool menu and by checking the Solver text box. After defining a linear model in a spreadsheet, the model can be solved directly by Solver, which generates two major reports: the solution report and the awareness (sensitivity) report. Solution reports give the solution and information/ status of constraints with slack values. An awareness report gives information about how sensitive the solution is. There are many advantages of using spread-sheets for ration formulation: it saves time and manpower, it gives less human error and it is easy to handle more amounts of feed ingredients and constraints effectively. In MS-Excel 2010, there are three methods available in the Solver tool, namely, the simplex method, generalized reduced gradient (GRG) nonlinear and the evolutionary algorithm (EA), which can be used to solve linear or nonlinear programming models.

DOI: 10.1201/9781003231714-3

3.1.1 Simplex LP Method in MS-Excel Solver

The simplex LP method is an iterative method which was developed by George Dantzig in 1946. According to the *Journal of Computing in Science and Technology* (Nash 2000), this method is considered one of the top ten algorithms. This method can be applied to solve a problem which has a first-degree equation (linear objective function) as well as linear constraints. In a plane, the linear function provides a straight line while plotting. The Excel Solver-based simplex method provides optimal results at the point where two or more constraints intersect, that is, the optimal result lies at the corner point.

To solve a linear programming problem (LPP) effectively by creating an ideal starting point, one has to check three basic requirements: a) the problem should be a maximization problem but can be converted to a minimization problem by rewriting the objective function with a minus sign; b) linear constraints must be less than or equal to an inequality; and c) all decision variables should be non-negative. The simplex LP method is an iterative process which is used to solve LPPs, has first degree equations and is applicable if all decision variables as well as constraints are linear functions. The LPP should have a clear representation of the linear relationship between constraints and variables; that is, if the variables of the LP model are bounded, then due to the rigidity of the problem, the LP simplex method fails to satisfy constraints.

3.1.2 GRG Nonlinear in MS-Excel Solver

The GRG method based on the work published by Leon Lasdon in 1973 and Alan Waren in 1975 is smooth. It deals with an equation involving decision variables or nonlinear constraints; that is, the derivative of the nonlinear function should not have any break point, and it should be continuous. If the graph of the function has a sharp point, it means that the derivative is discontinuous. In MS Excel 2010, the GRG algorithm picks a starting value from its calculation and hence leads to different answers on each run as it chooses a different starting point every time. The GRG method provides a global optimum solution if all functions and constraints are convex. If any function and constraints are non-convex, then it may get stuck in local optimum solutions. The GRG nonlinear strategy might be utilized to find the solution of any linear problem yet will do so substantially less effectively than the simplex LP technique. The GRG nonlinear is a proved reliable technique to solve nonlinear problems, but it can also work for LPPs. The technique takes a long time and is less efficient for LPPs but is preferable if the linear functions are rigid.

3.1.3 Evolutionary Algorithm in MS-Excel Solver

Evolutionary algorithm (EA) is a term used to portray a computer-based problem-solving tool which utilizes computational models as an important element to solve the problem whose functions or constraints are discontinuous and non-smooth. The MS-Excel-based evolutionary algorithm can obtain optimal solution only if the problem or model (LP or NLPP) is well scaled. An evolutionary algorithm does not depend on the derivative or gradient information; therefore, it is very difficult to determine at intermediate steps whether the result is optimal or not, and Solver stops with message like, "Solver Converged to Current Solution". This message indicates that the fitness of the current population of the trial solution is changing slowly, which means that Solver has found a global optimal solution. However, less diversity in the population is a very common problem in evolutionary algorithms, which indicates that EA fails to return a better solution through mutation, and it requires another important parameter like crossover to improve the diversity of the population. Solver also stops when it cannot improve the solution further; that is, even though EA spends enough (sometimes relatively more) time searching the better solution, if it fails to make progress, it will stop with the message "Best Solution Found". Therefore, once a solution is found using the Excel-based evolutionary algorithm, one can use these steps to improve the solution further (just a try): a) keep the generated solution and restart the solver with an EA option to see whether it is able to find a better answer in less time; b) reduce the convergence value and increase the maximum sub-problem and the maximum feasible value and restart the Solver; and c) an increase in population size as well as mutation rate can also help in finding the better solution, as an increase in mutation rate will increase the diversity of the population.

There are different varieties of EA, but MS Excel 2010 uses the basic algorithm, which starts with an initial random population for evaluating fitness. It only uses mutation as a parameter to improve the diversity of the population in every generation. In Chapter 5, the performance of the MS Excel-based Solver is discussed in detail by solving three different linear programming models of dairy cattle.

3.1.4 MATLAB (Matrix-Laboratory)

MATLAB is a license-based scientific package product of MathWorks; it is designed for easy and quick scientific calculation and graphic visualization in a high level programming language. MATLAB was originally written by MathWorks scientist Dr. Cleve Moler for easy matrix software developed in LINPACK and EISPACK projects. Its first version was written in the 1970s for course use in linear algebra, numerical analysis and matrix theory. Therefore, MATLAB is built with a foundation of matrix software where the input element (data) is a matrix which does not require pre-dimensioning. MATLAB has many inbuilt functions for a variety of computations; it also has many toolboxes designed for specific research fields, which include statistics, optimization, solution of ordinary and partial differential equation and data analysis. If anyone wants to use MATLAB for the first time in experimenting with genetic algorithms, a variety of inbuilt functions can be used. Problems can also be coded in m-files in a short time using these functions. In addition to this, a genetic algorithm can also be experimented with in a MATLAB-based toolbox called an optimization toolbox. The optimization toolbox is a collection of routines which is written in m-files, which implement the most useful functions in GA. GA is a heuristic-based search technique based on natural selection of the fittest, which is used to solve any sort of constrained as well as unconstrained optimization problem. GA starts with random number generation and then constantly modifies the population where, in every step, it randomly selects individuals from the present population and uses them as a parent to create new children for the next generation. After many generations the set of the population tends toward an optimal solution. There are many options and inbuilt functions in MATLAB to modify the parameters of the genetic algorithm according to the nature of the optimization problem. Genetic algorithm differs from old classical methods because old classical methods create only one point at every iterative step where a string of points approach the best-fit solution, whereas genetic algorithm creates a population at every iteration, and the best-fit individual approaches the optimal solution. In MATLAB using an inbuilt function, in general, genetic algorithm can be defined as follows:

3.1.4.1 *Inputs for Genetic Algorithm*

Number of Variables = []; Population Size = [];
Linear Inequalities of the form Ax=b
A = []; b = [];
Lower and Upper Bounds
Lower bound   = []; Upper bound = [];
ObjectiveFunction   = @ {specify the m-file of objective function};
Setting Options for
Genetic Algorithm
options   = gaoptimset.
options   = gaoptimset (options,'PopulationType',' {specify the function name}');
options   = gaoptimset (options,'CreationFcn', {specify the function name});
options   = gaoptimset (options,'PopulationSize', [specify the value]);
options   = gaoptimset (options,'EliteCount', [specify the value]);
options   = gaoptimset (options,'TolFun',[specify the value]);
options   = gaoptimset (options,'CrossoverFraction',[specify the value]);
options   = gaoptimset (options,'PopInitRange',[specify the range]);
options   = gaoptimset (options,'Generations',[specify the value]);
options   = gaoptimset (options,'StallGenLimit',[specify the value]);
options   = gaoptimset (options,'StallTimeLimit',[specify the value]);
options   = gaoptimset (options,'CrossoverFcn', {specify the function name});
options   = gaoptimset (options,'MutationFcn', { pecify the function name});
options   = gaoptimset (options,'SelectionFcn', {specify the function name});
options   = gaoptimset (options,'Display', '{specify the function name}');
options   = gaoptimset (options,'Display', '{specify the function name}');
options   = gaoptimset (options,'PlotFcns', specify the function name });
[x, fval]   = ga (ObjectiveFunction, numberOfVariables, A, b,[],[],lb,ub, [],options);
(https://in.mathworks.com/help/gads/genetic-algorithm/2016/.html)

Gaoptimset provides the options for GA parameters. Populace type represents the type of data in the population, and by default it takes "double vector". Creating an initial population is very important for the algorithm, as the entire population set is based on initial population; hence, the creation function creates the initial population in which "gacreationlinearfeasible" is the best option to create the initial population which satisfies all bounds as well as linear constraints. Therefore, we have created an initial population in the range of lower and upper bounds. The population size describes how many individuals should be there in each generation. Even though giving a large population size makes the algorithm run slowly, it is better to keep a large population size, as by keeping a large population size we are allowing an algorithm to search in a broader space and there is less chance for the algorithm to stop at local optima. Elite count describes the count of individuals that are assured to remain in every genesis; it takes only positive integers, or if the value is not assigned, it takes the default value as a ceiling (0.05 × population size). Elitism is very important in respect to convergence, as by allowing at least two or three individuals to survive at every generation, it makes the algorithm converge faster. Crossover is a very important parameter of the genetic algorithm as it combines two best-fit parents to create new offspring at every generation. "CrossoverFcn" options define the crossover type. There exist various kinds of crossover, such as 1-point crossover, 2-point crossover etc., but for linear constraints and bounds, "crossoverheuristic" is the best option for creating offspring. "Crossoverheuristic" returns offspring which lie on the line that involves two parents; one can specify how far the children is from the better parent by the parameter ratio. MATLAB takes the default value of this ratio as 1:2. In general, let P_1 and P_2 be the two parents and P_1 has high quality robust value, crossoverheuristic will return the offspring by the formula $P_2 + ratio \times (P_1 - P_2)$. The crossover fraction gives the division of each populace children that are other than world class children (elite children) which are comprised of crossover children. If the value of the crossover fraction is 1, it reveals that the algorithm is not having mutation, whereas if the crossover fraction is 0 it reflects that algorithm is running without crossover. Therefore, it is a good choice to keep the value of crossover fraction in between 0.6–0.8 for better diversity. Like crossover, mutation is also an important parameter of genetic algorithm to maintain the diversity of population; it allows the algorithm to search in a broader space. Mutation generally help the algorithm make small adjustments in an entity to create a mutation child. One can define the mutation option by the function name "MutationFcn". Due to rigidity in linear constraints, preference is given to "mutationadaptfeasible", where an adaptive feasible mutation generates a direction which is flexible compared to a previous lucrative or doomed genesis. This mutation chooses a direction and step length that satisfies both linear constraints as well as bounds. The selection operator helps the algorithm to select best-fit parents for the next generation; one can specify this option with the function name "selectionFcn". There are many types of selection procedures, such as roulette wheel selection, uniform selection etc., but preference is given to tournament selection, as the algorithm will choose each parent by its tournament size 2 at random, and then the best individual out of these will be selected as parent. Once these parameters are defined, the genetic algorithm Solver is called to run the program. These parameters can be tested on different types of optimization problems (linear or nonlinear), but these parameters need to be modified as per the requirements. In Chapters 5 and 6, the performance of this MATLAB-based genetic algorithm is tested on linear and nonlinear goal programming problems for least cost ration formulation (Kuntal et al., 2016).

3.2 Data Handling and Nutrient Bound Calculator

To formulate the ration problem, the following steps need to be followed: calculation of nutrient requirement, selection of ingredients, fixing the constraints and finding the result. These steps are discussed in detail in Chapters 5 and 6, where the calculation of the correct nutrients requirement for the specific body condition of cattle is first priority. The nutrient requirement of Indian dairy cattle and buffaloes is calculated as per the Indian Council of Agricultural Research (ICAR-NIANP, 2013) and National Research Council (NRC, 2001) standards. As discussed in Chapter 1, since 1957 much research has been done on calculating the nutritive value of Indian cattle. After many successive experiments, Kearl compiled the entire data on nutritional requirements of different livestock species, from which India come across a publication of nutrient requirement of cattle and buffalo in 1985. Since then many corrections have been done in the data, and finally ICAR came with another publication of nutrient requirements of cattle and buffalo in 2013. Therefore, to calculate the nutrient requirements, the primary data for the Mandya district of Karnataka is collected from (ICAR-NIANP), which is located in Adugodi, Bangalore.

An Excel-based nutrient bound calculator software for cattle and buffalo has been developed with the help of the Pr. Scientist of NIANP which is based on publication of nutrient requirements of cattle and buffalo (ICAR-NIANP, 2013) as well as NRC 2001 standards. The above-mentioned publication has all types of information which can be used for nutrient calculation as per the requirement.

4

Binary Coded Genetic Algorithm to Solve Ration Formulation Problem

CONTENTS

4.1 Introduction

The farmers of India hold a small number of dairy animals, in which cattle and buffalo are the main animals used for milk production. With the increase in the number of high milk producing dairy animals in different part of India due to many cross-breeding programs, there is a shortage of feed ingredients for dairy animals, due to which farmers are more conscious about scientific animal feeding practices. In addition to that, because of environmental hazards and global warming problems due to animal excreta, balancing nutrition production for proper health and excretion is required. Many qualified animal nutritionists are also finding difficulty in formulating the low-cost balanced ration for growing dairy animals at different body conditions. Even though linear programming is a good method for formulating least cost diet, it has many limitations, as the linear programming technique requires the objective function to be single and constraints to be rigid (RHS). Recently, many researchers have described the benefits of the goal programming method for ration formulation in which the weighted sum goal programming with a penalty function is used to solve the problem. In this research, an attempt is made to test the effectiveness of a heuristic algorithm such as a genetic algorithm to optimize the ration formulation on nonlinear and goal programming models.

DOI: 10.1201/9781003231714-4

4.2 Linear and Nonlinear Programming Model for Animal Feed Formulation (Test-Problem-1)

This research is primarily based on the secondary records of the linear and non-linear mathematical model of livestock ration formulation developed by Pratiksha Sexena (2011). This nonlinear model was developed for Sahiwal cows during the second to fifth lactation period, based on experimental data collected from National Dairy Research Institute (NDRI). Research was carried out on Sahiwal cows during second to fifth lactation period. It was divided into four categories that are replaced by four times in Latin-square change-over style. Every lactation period has a duration of 40 days. These divided categories, namely A, B, C and D, have been supplied with isonitrogenous as well as isocaloric concentrate mixtures which include groundnut and cotton seed cake individually (see Table 4.1). To fulfill the requirement of maintaining 50 grams of dicalcium phosphate (DCP), half of the quantity can be met through a concentrate mixture. A green fodder is added in order to provide the remaining DCP and to fulfill the dry matter and energy requirements. Other different concentrate mixtures which contain groundnut, cotton seed cake (undecorticated and decorticated) were also examined for crude protein, crude fiber, ether extract, organic waste, nitrogen free extract and total ash (Gupta et al., 2013b). This research work was based on the objective of maximizing the milk yield. Milk yields and production for which the nutrients are used predominantly rely upon three variables which might be utilized to amplify production (Gupta et al., 2013b). Keeping every one of these actualities, milk yield of an animal relies on digestible crude protein and total digestible nutrients.

4.2.1 Linear Programming Formulation

By using least square method, Pratiksha Sexena has developed a linear relationship between milk yield of cows and nutrient ingredients such as crude protein and TDN, which describes the weightage of variables x_1, x_2 and x_3. By using this

TABLE 4.1

Composition of Concentrate Mixtures in Respect of DCP and TDN

Ingredients	Control group (groundnut cake)	Cotton seed (whole)	Cotton seed cake (undecorticated)	Cotton seed cake (decorticated)
Groundnut cake	22	10	0	0
Cotton seed	0	57	0	0
(undecorticated)	0	0	44	0
(decorticated)	0	0	0	27
Wheat bran	75	30	53	70
Common salt	2	2	2	2
Mineral mixture	1	1	1	1

relationship, an objective function is formulated where the constraints are applied according to feeding standards of the National Research Council (NRC, 1981). The LP model is as follows:

$$\text{Maximize } y = 0.00403908701533x_1 + 0.25469485541324x_2 \\ + 0.02110699233x_3 - 8.67895696598672$$

$$\text{Subject to: } x_1 = (608.6718, 782.978), x_2 = (60.41, 75.943), x_3 \\ = (366.0412, 508.9343)$$

This LP model is solved by the simplex method, which leads to the solution as $x_1 = 782.97800$, $x_2 = 75.943$, $x_3 = 508.9343$ gm/kg metabolic body weight, with maximum objective value of 24.55.

4.2.2 Nonlinear Programming Formulation

Pratiksha Sexena further developed a relationship between y and x_1, y and x_2, y and x_3 by using the least square method and by using different degrees (F-test) to find the relation of best fit. Hence, a nonlinear objective function is formulated mathematically with the relation of variables as per their weightage on milk production, where the constraints are incorporated as per NRC (1981) standards. The nonlinear model is as follows:

$$y = 4.1792442x_2^2 - 4.082239204 * 10^{-6}x_3^2 + 0.114836671x_1 - 560.0786654x_2 \\ + 4.145857585 * 10^{-3}x_3 + 19255.68675. - (1)$$

Subject to:
$$x_1 = (608.6718, 782.978), x_2 = (60.641, 75.943), x_3 = (366.0412, 508.9343)$$

This nonlinear model is solved by using the Kuhn-Tucker method, which gives the values of the three nutrient ingredients as $x_1 = (782.97800)$, $x_2 = (67.00717)$, $x_3 = (507.79209)$ gm/kg metabolic body weight, with a maximum objective value of 582.01 gm/kg metabolic weight.

4.2.3 Extended Work Using Genetic Algorithms

In the present study an attempt is made to study the effect of a binary genetic algorithm over a nonlinear model described by Pratiksha Sexena. The study further extends the importance of nonlinear livestock ration formulation and finds its solution by another heuristic approach called controlled random search technique (RST2, Gupta and Chandan, 2013). Both the genetic algorithm (GA) and RST2 are heuristic and random search techniques with the most important features of function evaluation. Briefly, RST2 was developed by C. Mohan and Shankar (1994) based on random number generation; it does not consider the mathematical nature of the function and still gives promising results. RST2 is an iterative process which works on the principle of quadratic approximation. It works in two phases, namely a local as well as a global phase, without making any prior assumptions about the objective function or constraints. In the global phase, an objective function is estimated at random based on sample feasible points, and in the local phase, these feasible points are controlled by local search options to produce a best fit individual for global minima. GA is an optimization method which is used to optimize both constrained and unconstrained optimization problems; it is an adaptive heuristic algorithm which works on Darwin's principle of survival of the fittest. The idea behind genetic algorithm is to simulate the process in the natural system which is necessary for evolution. GA not only provides an alternative method but also outperforms the other traditional methods consistently. GA starts with set of solutions (chromosomes) called the population. Solution from one set of population has been taken to create a new set of population with the hope that the new set of population is better than the old one. This new set of solutions (offspring) will be chosen from the population based on its best fitness value. The robust value is allocated to every individual, where computation of robust value depends upon the application. At every iteration (generations), candidates are chosen from the set of randomly generated population for reproduction of new offspring by crossover and mutation, where crossover will be done with high probability compared to mutation. The selection of individuals will be depending upon high fitness, but the mean fitness of population likes to improve the solution from generation to generation. Due to its random nature, GA improves the chance of finding the global optimum solution. We have slightly modified the technique to suit our requirements and solved the nonlinear programming problem described by Pratiksha Sexena.

4.2.4 Solution of Nonlinear Programming Model by Genetic Algorithm

A result of the nonlinear model solved by GA for original bounds Test Problem-1) is given in Table 4.2, from which the set of solutions obtained are: $x_1 = (721.3220, 747.1494)$, $x_2 = (71.5456, 74.6055)$, $x_3 = (432.318, 474.6072)$, with the global maxima of 819.1805. Sometimes due to random numbers generated initially and huge intervals, solutions seem to be stuck in the local optimum. Therefore, to avoid this we have reduced the bounds as follows: $x_1 = (630.682)$; $x_2 = (66.70)$; $x_3 = (366.480)$ (Test Problem-2). The set of solutions for NLP model (2) by GA for the reduced bounds are given in Table 4.3. The set of solutions obtained are $x_1 = (670.5081, 677.1270)$, $x_2 = (68.8769, 69.4029)$, $x_3 = (428.7671, 463.4859)$ with the global maxima of 593.8254. Also, the comparison result of RST2 and GA is given in Table 4.4.

TABLE 4.2

Solution for NLP Model by GA for Original Bounds (Test Problem-1)

Iterations	x_1 (gm/kg metabolic weight)	x_2 (gm/kg metabolic weight)	x_3 (gm/kg metabolic weight)	Objective function
100	749.0624	73.5973	432.3138	759.5984
200	755.6987	72.4891	495.7266	704.4718
300	744.6752	74.2517	491.5240	796.9501
400	729.9346	72.8592	457.8180	719.0342
500	750.7326	73.6261	475.2268	761.3943

Iterations	x_1 (gm/kg metabolic weight)	x_2 (gm/kg metabolic weight)	x_3 (gm/kg metabolic weight)	Objective function
600	747.5276	71.5456	472.9012	664.0140
700	748.0788	72.9356	463.3000	724.8789
800	721.3220	72.9743	465.8431	723.7324
900	759.4326	73.2797	482.3860	743.7354
1000	724.1868	73.1996	484.8339	735.5141
2000	722.4416	72.5642	482.3343	704.1149
3000	747.1494	74.6055	474.6072	819.1805
4000	724.4928	74.5268	472.6285	811.6016
5000	759.6734	73.2089	477.6959	740.0712

TABLE 4.3

Solution for NLP Model by GA for Reduced Bounds (Test Problem-2)

Iterations	x_1 (gm/kg metabolic weight)	x_2 (gm/kg metabolic weight)	x_3 (gm/kg metabolic weight)	Objective function
100	672.1468	69.3301	463.4448	591.8256
200	672.0984	68.8769	428.7671	583.8616
300	664.0533	69.3305	439.3848	590.8939
400	662.9170	68.8893	456.7290	583.0166
500	677.1270	69.4029	445.7669	593.8254
600	670.5509	69.4217	444.8161	593.4490
700	662.0822	69.4115	463.4859	592.2789
800	672.0792	69.3436	446.4769	592.0740
900	669.2510	69.1619	460.0039	588.3455
1000	674.4207	69.0258	461.6140	586.5650
2000	674.7802	69.3380	456.8179	592.2804
3000	662.8439	69.0090	453.2494	584.9496
4000	675.4472	69.3782	441.0744	593.1386
5000	670.5081	69.1511	442.2030	588.2859

TABLE 4.4

Comparison of Solution Obtained by GA and RST for NLP Model

Bounds	RST2				GA			
	x_1	x_2	x_3	Obj. func.	x_1	x_2	x_3	Obj. func.
Original bounds	608–680	66–68	400–512	562–569.9	721.32–747.14	71.54–74.60	432.31–474.60	664–819.18
Reduced bounds	630–642	66.82–67.22	380–438.5	564–566	670.5–677.12	68.87–69.40	428.76–463.48	583–593.82

4.2.5 Graphical Results

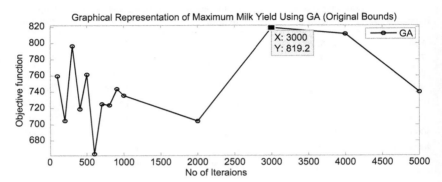

FIGURE 4.1 Maximum Milk Yield Using GA (Original Bounds); Kuntal, IJESET, 2003.

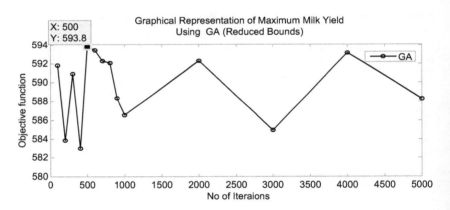

FIGURE 4.2 Maximum Milk Yield Using GA (Reduced Bounds), Kuntal, IJESET, 2003

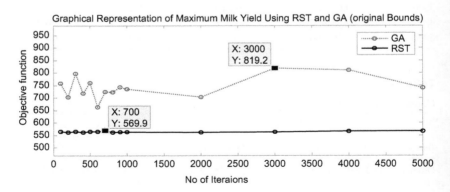

FIGURE 4.3 Maximum Milk Yield Using RST and GA (Original Bounds), Kuntal, IJESET, 2003

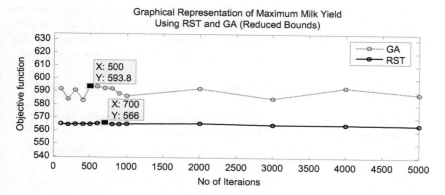

FIGURE 4.4 Maximum Milk Yield Using RST and GA (Reduced Bounds), Kuntal, IJESET, 2003

4.3 Goal-Programming Model (Test Problem-2)

This study is extracted from the work of Shrabani Gosh (2011), with an objective of studying the effectiveness of GA over the goal programming (GP) model of the ration formulation problem. Briefly, farmers encountered three circumstances for a fully grown cow with a body weight of 500 kg: a) cow did not produce milk; b) cow produces various levels of milk with a specific percentage of fat; c) cow is pregnant at third trimester, where it requires an extra nutrient supplement.

Therefore, farmers need to feed a low-cost balanced ration to all of these categories. Based on these three categories, a linear programming model for animal-1, animal-2 and animal-3 has been developed where animal-1 needs a ration only for body maintenance, animal-2 needs a ration for body maintenance as well as for 10 litres of milk production with 4% fat and animal-3 needs a ration for third trimester pregnancy. Nutrient requirements as well as the constraints for all three categories were set as per the Indian Council of Agricultural Research (ICAR) standard (Ranjan, 1998) and as per Mondal et al. (2003). These LP models are solved using the simplex method. Further, to overcome the limitations of the LP model, a linear goal programming model for three categories of animal has been developed and solved by simplex method. Since Shrabani formulated the global linear model, in the extension of this a nonlinear GP model was developed by taking the square root of sum of the squares of the deviations in which the weight is attached to every goal as per the priority.

4.3.1 Formulation of the Nonlinear Goal Programming Problem

The general GP model is as follows: $\text{Min}(Z) = \Sigma_{i \in m} p_i(d_i^+ + d_i^-)$, subjected to $\sum_{j=1}^{n}(a_{ij}x_j + d_i^- - d_i^+) = g_i$, where $d_i^-, d_i^+, x_j \geq 0$ and $(i = 1,2 \dots m)$ and $(j = 1,2, \dots n)$; d_i^+, d_i^- represents the +*ve* and −*ve* deviational variable, which needs to overachieve and underachieve the ith goal; x_j represents the decision variables; a_{ij} represents the coefficients of the decision variable; p_i represents the level of priority which is assigned to every goal. In this nonlinear GP model with nonlinear objective function (Gupta et al., 2013b), goals are allotted in such a fashion that all +ve deviational variables (≤), −ve deviational variables (≥) and both +ve and −ve deviational variables (=) need to be minimized. The brief description of the goals requirements is as follows:

G-1: d_{lc}^-, d_{lc}^+ represent an under- and overachievement of least cost ration, where d_{lc}^+ requires minimization.

G-2 and 3: d_t^-, d_t^+ represent under- and overachievement of total weight of feed ingredients, where both require minimization.

G-4: d_{cp}^- and d_{cp}^+ represent under- and overachievement of the protein requirement, where d_{cp}^- requires minimization.

G-5: d_{tdn}^- and d_{tdn}^+ represent under- and overachievement of the energy requirement, in which d_{tdn}^- requires minimization.

G-6: d_{ca}^- and d_{ca}^+ represent under- and overachievement of the calcium requirement, where d_{ca}^- requires minimization.

G-7: d_p^- and d_p^+ represent under- and overachievement of the phosphorus requirement, where d_p^- requires minimization.

G-8: d_g^- and d_g^+ represent under- and overachievement of the grain, maize and jowar requirement, where d_g^+ requires minimization.

G-9: d_b^- and d_b^+ represent under- and overachievement of the bran rice and wheat requirement, in which d_b^+ requires minimization.

G-10: d_{ck}^- and d_{ck}^+ represent under- and overachievement of the groundnut cake as well as the cotton cake requirement, where d_{ck}^+ requires minimization.

G-11 and 12: $d_{r/c}^-$ and $d_{r/c}^+$ give under- and over-achievement of roughage as well as concentrate ratio (that is, 2:3), where both the deviations require minimization.

G-13 and 14: $d_{d/g}^-$ and $d_{d/g}^+$ represent under- and overachievement of dry-green ratio (that is, 2:3), where both the deviations need to be minimized.

G-15 and 16: $d_{c/h}^-$ and $d_{c/h}^+$ represent the under- and overachievement ratio of legume and non-legume (that is, cowpea: hybrid Napier in ratio of 1:1), where both the deviations require minimization. The GP model is nonlinear, as the objective function involves the square root of the sum of the squares of the deviations, in which the weight is allocated to every goal as per the priority (Gupta et al., 2013b). The goal programming model has 12 goals and nine decision variables, with 24 deviational variables. The objective function has been formulated by considering deviational variables for each goal (maximization or minimization) whose target is given on RHS. The nonlinear GP model for all three levels of animals is given in Table 4.5 where,

1. $P_1 \ldots {}_{16}$ in the objective function indicates goals set as per priorities, x_1 = Paddy, x_2 = Hybrid Napier, x_3 = Cowpea, x_4 = Maize grain, x_5 = Jowar grain, x_6 = Rice bran, x_7 = Wheat bran, x_8 = Groundnut cake, x_9 = Cotton seed cake
2. P (lc, t, cp, TDN, Ca, p, c, b, CK, r/c, d/g, c/h)$^-$, P (lc, t, cp, TDN, Ca, p, c, b, CK, r/c, d/g, c/h)$^+$ indicates positive and negative deviation
3. $x_1 \ldots {}_9 \geq 0$, P (lc, t, cp, TDN, Ca, p, c, b, CK, r/c, d/g, c/h) ≥ 0 (Tables 4.6–4.8)

TABLE 4.5

Nonlinear GP Model with Priority Ranked Goals for Animal at Level-1 to 3 with Objective Function (z) to Different Goals Which Need to Be Minimized

$$\text{Min}(z) = \sqrt{\begin{array}{l} P_1 d_{lc}^{+2} + P_2 d_t^{-2} + P_3 d_t^{+2} + P_4 d_{cp}^{+2} + P_5 d_{tdn}^{-2} + P_6 d_{ca}^{-2} + P_7 d_p^{-2} + P_8 d_g^{+2} + P_9 d_b^{+2} + P_{10} d_{ck}^{+2} + P_{11} d_{\frac{r}{c}}^{-2} \\ + P_{12} d_{\frac{r}{c}}^{+2} + P_{13} d_{\frac{d}{g}}^{-2} + P_{14} d_{\frac{d}{g}}^{+2} + P_{15} d_{\frac{c}{h}}^{-2} + P_{16} d_{\frac{c}{h}}^{+2} \end{array}}$$

Subjected to constraints	Level-1	Level-2	Level-3
Least cost (Rs/kg):	≤7.48	≤9.01	≤8.17
$4x_1 + 2x_2 + 4x_3 + 10x_4 + 9x_5 + 12x_6 + 12x_7 + 14x_8 + 20x_9 + d_{lc}^- - d_{lc}^+$			
Total (kg): $x_1 + x_2 + x_3 + x_4 + x_5 + x_6 + x_7 + x_8 + x_9 + d_t^- - d_t^+$	= 1	= 1	= 1
Protein (g/kg):	≥31	≥108	≥46.53
$30x_1 + 10x_2 + 180x_3 + 80x_4 + 110x_5 + 120x_6 + 120x_7 + 450x_8 + 300x_9 + d_{CP}^- - d_{CP}^+$			
TDN/Energy (g/kg):	≥297	≥693	≥445
$4540x_1 + 550x_2 + 600x_3 + 880x_4 + 850x_5 + 660x_6 + 650x_7 + 790x_8 + 790x_9 + d_{TDN}^- - d_{TDN}^+$			
Calcium (g/kg):	≥3.8	≥5.15	≥3.1
$2x_1 + 5.6\,x_2 + 12.8\,x_3 + 2.7\,x_4 + 3\,x_5 + 2.4\,x_6 + 2.6\,x_7 + 3.8\,x_8 + 7.4\,x_9 + d_{Ca}^- - d_{Ca}^+$			
Phosphorus (g/kg):	≥2.3	≥3.78	≥2.3
$1.1x_1 + 3.8\,x_2 + 5.7\,x_3 + 4.2\,x_4 + 3.9\,x_5 + 17.3\,x_6 + 13.7\,x_7 + 8.4\,x_8 + 13.9\,x_9 + d_P^- - d_P^+$			
Grain max @ 70% of concentrate (kg): $x_4 + x_5 + d_g^- - d_g^+$	≤0.36	≤0.36	≤0.36
Bran max @ 50% of concentrate (kg): $x_6 + x_7 + d_b^- - d_b^+$	≤0.30	≤0.30	≤0.30
Cake max @ 30% of concentrate (kg): $x_8 + x_9 + d_{CK}^- - d_{CK}^+$	≤0.21	≤0.21	≤0.21
Roughage /concentrate: $3(x_1 + x_2 + x_3) - 2(x_4 + x_5 + x_6 + x_7 + x_8) + d_{r/c}^- - d_{r/c}^+$	= 0	= 0	= 0
Dry/green roughages: $3x_1 - 2(x_2 + x_3) + d_{d/g}^- - d_{d/g}^+$	= 0	= 0	= 0
Legume/non-legume greens: $x_2 - x_3 + d_{c/h}^- - d_{c/h}^+$	= 0	= 0	= 0

TABLE 4.6

Solution Set of LPP for Level-1, 2 and 3 by GA

Generation	Levels	x_1	x_2	x_3	x_4	x_5	x_6	x_7	x_8	x_9	Z
100	L-1	0.1174	0.0465	0.1002	0	0.2384	0	0.2627	0	0	0.2784
	L-2	0.0819	0.0638	0.0813	0	0.3225	0	0.0278	0	0.1	0.0134
	L-3	0.0649	0.0396	0.0422	0	0.3142	0	0.2633	0	0	0.5578
200	L-1	0.0678	0.0429	0.0718	0	0.3336	0	0.2201	0	0	0.2861
	L-2	0.064	0.0367	0.0959	0	0.3338	0	0.0155	0	0.0623	0.0149
	L-3	0.093	0.0381	0.0995	0	0.2960	0	0.2378	0	0.0000	0.586
300	L-1	0.0664	0.0289	0.1258	0	0.3253	0	0.2831	0	0	0.2814
	L-2	0.0599	0.0394	0.0516	0	0.3175	0	0.0228	0	0.1155	0.0159
	L-3	0.0775	0.0518	0.0857	0	0.2855	0	0.2477	0	0	0.6303
400	L-1	0.0756	0.0327	0.0741	0	0.2387	0	0.2286	0	0	0.2656
	L-2	0.0834	0.0509	0.0648	0	0.3389	0	0.0312	0	0.0539	0.0102
	L-3	0.0930	0.0381	0.0995	0	0.2960	0	0.2378	0	0	0.5860
500	L-1	0.1039	0.0311	0.0758	0	0.2815	0	0.2605	0	0	0.2852
	L-2	0.0534	0.0538	0.1118	0	0.3261	0	0.0194	0	0.0849	0.0136
	L-3	0.0378	0.0299	0.1477	0	0.2983	0	0.2648	0	0	0.6098
600	L-1	0.1027	0.0362	0.0943	0	0.3287	0	0.2692	0	0	0.2767
	L-2	0.1106	0.0547	0.0655	0	0.3572	0	0.0269	0	0.0957	0.0113
	L-3	0.0903	0.0428	0.1197	0	0.3174	0	0.2262	0	0	0.6064
700	L-1	0.0961	0.0289	0.0683	0	0.2651	0	0.2309	0	0	0.2782
	L-2	0.0803	0.0507	0.1096	0	0.2991	0	0.017	0	0.1074	0.0119
	L-3	0.1154	0.0427	0.0837	0	0.3460	0	0.2506	0	0	0.6247
800	L-1	0.0873	0.0486	0.152	0	0.2806	0	0.2371	0	0	0.2629
	L-2	0.1191	0.0524	0.0752	0	0.3464	0	0.0285	0	0.0612	0.0183
	L-3	0.0857	0.0379	0.1244	0	0.2960	0	0.2427	0	0	0.5931
900	L-1	0.0667	0.0486	0.0889	0	0.3224	0	0.2772	0	0	0.2864
	L-2	0.0700	0.0713	0.0983	0	0.3084	0	0.0182	0	0.0623	0.0116
	L-3	0.0311	0.0461	0.0794	0	0.3150	0	0.2284	0	0	0.6406
1000	L-1	0.072	0.1931	0.0000	0	0.2161	0	0.1529	0	0.0230	0.2014
	L-2	0.1028	0.0545	0.0876	0	0.3411	0	0.0237	0	0	0.0167
	L-3	0.1134	0.0326	.096	0	.2928	0	.2767	0	0	.4880

Solution Set of the Nonlinear Programming Problem (NLPP) for Level-1, 2 and 3 by GA

Generations	Levels	x_1	x_2	x_3	x_4	x_5	x_6	x_7	x_8	x_9	Z
100	L-1	0.0997	0.1663	0	0	0.246	0	0.145	0	0	0.174
	L-2	0.1334	0.0589	0.0786	0	0.356	0	0.026	0	0.097	0.022
	L-3	0.0507	0.035	0.0926	0	0.342	0	0.262	0	0	0.528
200	L-1	0.0555	0.1887	0	0	0.253	0	0.132	0	0	0.164
	L-2	0.0641	0.0709	0.1129	0	0.352	0	0.024	0	0.089	0.027
	L-3	0.0601	0.0415	0.1002	0	0.277	0	0.265	0	0	0.499
300	L-1	0.0937	0.1617	0	0	0.231	0	0.197	0	0	0.166
	L-2	0.063	0.0688	0.1222	0	0.352	0	0.018	0	0.076	0.020
	L-3	0.0872	0.0416	0.0825	0	0.261	0	0.248	0	0	0.466
400	L-1	0.0993	0.2019	0	0	0.215	0	0.134	0	0	0.169
	L-2	0.1012	0.0544	0.0499	0	0.295	0	0.026	0	0.069	0.027
	L-3	0.0859	0.0444	0.0466	0	0.326	0	0.249	0	0	0.511
500	L-1	0.1078	0.1863	0	0	0.217	0	0.177	0	0	0.168
	L-2	0.0634	0.0685	0.0807	0	0.285	0	0.019	0	0.037	0.025
	L-3	0.1182	0.0428	0.0476	0	0.256	0	0.257	0	0	0.538
600	L-1	0.0926	0.1887	0	0	0.278	0	0.193	0	0	0.176
	L-2	0.1043	0.0809	0.1079	0	0.329	0	0.029	0	0.102	0.028
	L-3	0.1144	0.0463	0.0846	0	0.341	0	0.268	0	0	0.535
700	L-1	0.0677	0.1597	0	0	0.219	0	0.200	0	0	0.199
	L-2	0.0551	0.0469	0.113	0	0.335	0	0.028	0	0.071	0.023
	L-3	0.0821	0.0517	0.1025	0	0.252	0	0.263	0	0	0.556
800	L-1	0.0360	0.1712	0	0	0.227	0	0.161	0	0	0.187
	L-2	0.1227	0.0626	0.1185	0	0.374	0	0.026	0	0.086	0.029
	L-3	0.087	0.0303	0.0938	0	0.312	0	0.239	0	0	0.563
900	L-1	0.1273	0.1365	0	0	0.194	0	0.179	0	0	0.178
	L-2	0.1248	0.0746	0.1132	0	0.346	0	0.018	0	0.054	0.027
	L-3	0.0768	0.0368	0.0492	0	0.328	0	0.250	0	0	0.532
1000	L-1	0.1100	0.1518	0	0	0.256	0	0.203	0	0	0.179
	L-2	0.0531	0.0553	0.0805	0	0.254	0	0.025	0	0.041	0.027
	L-3	0.0903	0.0328	0.0863	0	0.289	0	0.273	0	0	0.552

TABLE 4.8

Comparison of Decision Variables by RST and GA

Variable	GA			RST		
	L-1	L-2	L-3	L-1	L-2	L-3
x_1	0.036–0.127	0.0531–0.1334	0.0507–0.1182	0.1–0.196	0.102–0.146	0.102–0.158
x_2	0.137–0.2019	0.0469–0.0809	0.0303–0.0517	0.101–0.216	0.027–0.068	0.055–0.077
x_3	0–0	0.0499–0.1185	0.0466–0.1025	0.017–0.084	0.141–0.153	0.150–0.187
x_4	0–0	0–0	0–0	0.052–0.088	0.062–0.076	0.055–0.098
x_5	0.1936–0.2559	0.2536–0.3737	0.2517–0.3421	0.309–0.386	0.314–0.389	0.301–0.395
x_6	0–0	0–0	0–0	0.050–0.068	0.059–0.086	0.057–0.095
x_7	0.1319–0.2026	0.0177–0.0286	0.2727–0.2685	0.204–0.318	0.012–0.047	0.201–0.299
x_8	0–0	0–0	0–0	0.059–0.089	0.050–0.087	0.050–0.088
x_9	0–0	0.0409–0.0964	0–0	0.050–0.088	0.101–0.153	0.50–0.649

4.3.2 Graphical Results

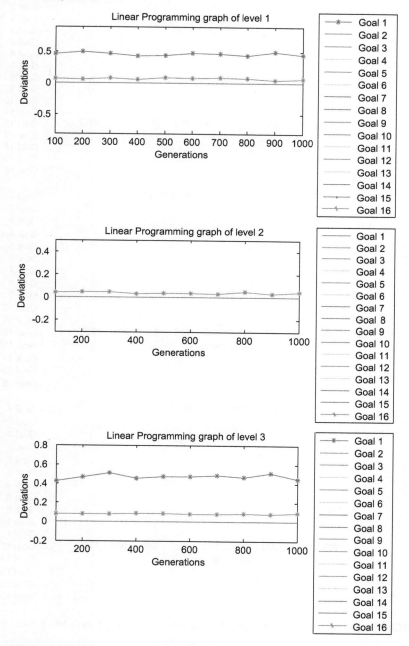

FIGURE 4.5 Graphs of Deviations for Linear Model of Level-1, 2 and 3, Kuntal, IJEIT, 2013.

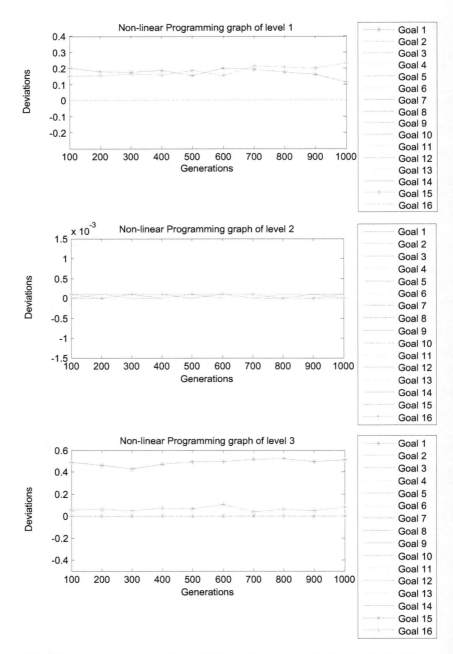

FIGURE 4.6   Deviations for Nonlinear GP Model of Level-1, 2 and 3, Kuntal, IJEIT, 2013

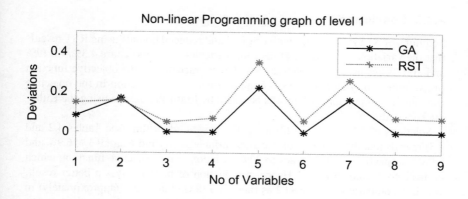

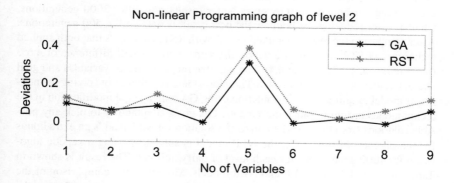

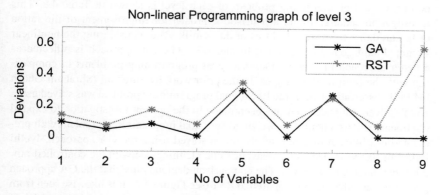

FIGURE 4.7   Comparison of GA and RST, Kuntal, IJEIT, 2013

4.3.3 Conclusion

Solutions of NLPP (1) and (2) with original and reduced bounds using RST reveals that the variation in the value of decision variables x_1, x_2 and x_3 are 4.3%, −0.19% and 20.17% respectively, which leads to 0.68% variation in the objective function (maximum milk yield). There is an approximately 2% deviation in the objective function in comparison with results obtained by Pratiksha Sexena using the Kuhn-Tucker condition.

Solutions of NLPP (1) and (2) using the genetic algorithm (see Tables 4.2 and 4.3) reveals that the variation of decision variables x_1, x_2 and x_3 are 9.3%, 6.9% and 6.08%, respectively, which leads to 27% variation in the objective function, which is more compared to RST2. Hence, a reduction of bounds gives a better result, which is comparable with RST2 as there is a deviation of 2% (approximately) in the objective function with the value obtained by the Kuhn-Tucker method. Using a wide range of bounds for GA gives better results only after 3000 generations, whereas after reducing the bounds, the best result is obtained in 500 generations. After comparing the results obtained by GA with RST2, it reveals that both applied techniques (RST2 and GA) are nearly the same, with a small difference of 4.6% (See Figures 4.1, 4.2, 4.3 and 4.4). The possible range of choice variables and goal characteristics is given in Table 4.4. Therefore, there is a chance of solving the nonlinear model of animal feed formulation using GA with a slight modification in the technique according to our requirements. GA gives adaptability to pick any possible solutions from the vast domain of the solution set, which adds an extra bonus for the planner. In this study, the NLP model is solved by using a genetic algorithm for 1000 generations for each level of dairy animals. The result is shown in Tables 4.6 and 4.7 for the LP and NLP models. Moreover, the comparison of the controlled random search technique (RST) and the genetic algorithm (GA) for the nonlinear goal programming problem of each level is shown in Table 4.8. This investigation centers around a heuristic approach for improvement of the ration of Indian dairy cows with 10 litres of daily milk yield, considering the nonlinear weighted sum goal programming formulation. The GA approach is reflected as a better approach in solving nonlinear goal programming problems in comparison with the prior methodologies. In the prior work by Shrabani (Shrabani Ghosh [M.Phil. dissertation] 2011) the linear goal programming problem was solved using Excel Solver. An endeavour has been made in the present investigation to expand the linear GPP as a nonlinear weighted sum goal programming problem with predefined priorities at different levels and is solved using the GA approach. Jyothi Lakshmi likewise made an endeavour to tackle this issue with the controlled random search technique (RST). The comparison demonstrates that the GA approach gives a better outcome as compared to RST (see Figure 4.7). It is likewise seen from the outcomes appeared in Table 4.6 that Goal-1 is overachieved by 46% to 50% of variation and Goal-15 is overachieved by 5% to 8.5% of variation for Level-1. In Level-2, Goal-16 is overachieved by 3.2% to 4.7% of variation. Also, in Level-3 Goal-1 is overachieved by 42.6% to 50.9% of variation. All other goals are achieved in a thousand generations using GA for the linear model. Figure 4.5 can be alluded to to see the wholistic perspective of the goal achievements. From Figure 4.6 we can observe that Goal-1 is overachieved by 16.2% to 20.2% and Goal-15 is overachieved by 14.9% to 21.3% of variation for Level-1. For Level-2, all the goals are achieved, and for Level-3, Goal-1 is overachieved by 46% to 51.8% and Goal-16 is overachieved by 5% to 10% of variation. All other goals are almost achieved in 1000 generations using GA for the NLP model. Thus, by considering these outcomes for the LP model, our tool gives more proficient rations by tweaking the nutritive goals and by taking innocuous deviations into consideration by treating them as underachievement and overachievement. The connected approach of the nonlinear weighted goal programming problem ends up being a helpful "motor" to formulate the least cost ration without any nutritive deficiency, which is the basic downside of the LP. The proficient ration can be improved further by adjusting the target values of the goals, but this tool may be useful for the assessment of consequences due to globalization impacts (input price rise, price volatility and environmental as well as climate change aspects).

5

Least Cost Feed Formulation for Dairy Cattle during Pregnancy by Using Real Coded Genetic Algorithm

An Application

CONTENTS

5.1 Introduction

In the Mandya district of Karnataka, dairy farmers have limited feedstuffs. Therefore, to fulfill nutrient requirements in terms of crude protein (CP), total digestible nutrients (TDN), calcium (Ca) and phosphorus (P), it was necessary to adopt a software program. There are many techniques/software that were adopted to fulfill the nutrient requirements of dairy animals (www.scialert.net); however, there is no specific technique suitable for formulating least cost rations for dairy animals. Hence, a comparative study was planned to find a suitable technique which is farmer friendly and can be used at the dairy farm level. The focus of this chapter is to provide a least cost diet formulation based on the nutrient

DOI: 10.1201/9781003231714-5

requirements of cattle which has been calculated according to the Indian Council of Agricultural Research (ICAR-NIANP, 2013) and National Research Council (NRC, 2001) standards during the third trimester of pregnancy. A linear programming model (LP) was formulated for three different types of cattle with body weight of 500 kg each and the requirement of a 10-litre milk yield with 4% of fat content, based on the seventh, eighth and ninth months of pregnancy on a dry matter basis. The LP model has been solved by a general reduced gradient (GRG) nonlinear, an evolutionary algorithm (EA), a simplex LP method and a real coded genetic algorithm (RGA) with and without seeding the random number generations. As far as the profit is concerned for the farmers, the cost of the feed plays an important role.

In 1951, Waugh applied linear programming technique developed by Koopmans (Waugh, 1951) to provide the solution of least cost dairy feed. Therefore, for the past seven decades conventional linear programming method was very popular to solve animal diet problems (Rehman, 1984; Oladokun and Johnson, 2012). In 2001, Tozer applied a multiple-objective technique to minimize the nutrient excretion from dairy cows through incorporation of a nutrient excretion function into ration formulation. In 2002, Zhang also applied multiple-objective programming to the feed formulation of a broiler grower ration with the objective of minimizing the nutrient variance and minimizing the ration cost. Many researchers have introduced the use of computer software and Excel Solver for solving linear programming problems (Folayan et al., 2008; Zgajnar et al., 2009; Sebastian et al., 2008; Radhika and Rao, 2010). Solving diet problems using the LP model mathematically only deals with primary technical issues, which can have a weak relationship with the commercial complication of reducing or increasing the change between costs and feeding over time. To overcome this problem various types of methodologies such as goal programming, multi-objective programming, nonlinear programming etc. have been used for many years (Rehman and Romero, 1984, 1987; Hertzler, 1987; Afrouziyeh et al., 2010; Saxena, 2011a). It has been shown that the linear programming approach indicates how best to combine available local ingredients effectively to formulate the least cost ration for broilers (Al-Deseit, 2009). Ghosh in 2014 combined LP with goal programming (GP) for feed formulation, displaying the dip in cost as a major advantage of using the goal-programming approach (Ghosh et al., 2014).

5.1.1 Data Collection and Methodology

The present work is based on primary data collected from the Mandya district of Karnataka as per ICAR-NIANP 2013 and NRC 2001 standards (ICAR-NIANP, 2013). Briefly, the cows during the third trimester of pregnancy need a balanced ration for body maintenance, milk production (with a minimum of 4% of fat content) and fetus growth. Therefore, to formulate the low-cost diet for these cows is a major challenge for farmers. So we have introduced LP models at three different months of pregnancy for different body weights. As the growth of the fetus increases significantly after six months of pregnancy, the nutrient requirements of cattle at the seventh, eighth and ninth month of pregnancy are presented in Tables 5.1 and 5.2. The estimation of nutrient requirements during late pregnancy requires accurate values for rates of nutrient accretion in conceptus tissues (ICAR-NIANP, 2013). The ration was formulated using the following steps:

Step-1 (calculation of nutrient requirement): The nutrient requirements of Cattle-, 2, and 3 are calculated based on body weight, milk yield, fat percentage and pregnancy status. Dry matter intake, crude protein and total digestible nutrients are calculated according to ICAR-NIANP 2013, phosphorus and calcium according to NRC 2001 standards on a dry matter basis (Table 5.1). Different categories of cattle are considered as follows:

TABLE 5.1

Nutrient Requirements of Cattle-1, 2 and 3

Level	Body weight (kg)	Milk yield (in litres)	Fat %	Pregnancy (in months)
Cattle 1	500	10	4	7
Cattle 2	500	10	4	8
Cattle 3	500	10	4	9

Step-2 (selection of ingredients): Based on primary data collected in the Mandya district of Karnataka, locally available roughages, concentrate and minerals are listed in Table 5.2. Among these ingredients, commonly available dry roughages are paddy straw and Ragi straw. Commonly available green roughages are Bajra X Napier grass (Co-4), multi-cut sorghum (Co-FS 29) and maize fodder. The nutrient content of the feed stuffs is shown in Table 5.2, and nutrient contents of feedstuffs are shown in Table 5.3.

TABLE 5.2

Selected Feedstuffs

Roughages	Concentrates	Minerals
Paddy straw	Maize	Calcite
Bajra X Napier Co-4 grass	Soya de-oiled cake (DOC)	Mineral mixture (MM)
Maize fodder	Copra DOC	Dicalcium phosphate (DCP)
Co-FS 29 sorghum	Cotton DOC	Salt
Ragi straw	Wheat bran	
	Gram chunnies	
	Cotton seed	
	Concentrate mix Type-1	

TABLE 5.3

Nutrient Content of Feedstuffs on DM basis

Feeds	DM (%)	CP (kg)	TDN (kg)	Ca (kg)	P (kg)	Cost (Rs)
Roughage						
Paddy straw	90	0.0513	0.4	0.0018	0.0008	5
Co-4 grass	25	0.08	0.52	0.00144	0.0009	3
Maize fodder	25	0.08	0.6	0.0053	0.0014	3
Co-FS 29 sorghum	90	0.07	0.5	0.0012	0.0009	3
Ragi straw	90	0.06	0.42	0.0015	0.0009	3
Concentrates						
Maize	90	0.081	0.792	0.00018	0.0027	17
Soya DOC	90	0.42	0.7	0.00018	0.00225	38
Copra DOC	90	0.22	0.7	0.00036	0.009	23
Cotton DOC	90	0.32	0.7	0.00036	0.009	23
Wheat bran	90	0.12	0.7	0.01067	0.00093	17
Gram chunnies	90	0.17	0.6	0.000108	0.00234	12
Cotton seed	90	0.16	1.1	0.003	0.0062	21
Conc. mix Type-I	90	0.22	0.7	0.005	0.0045	17
Calcite	97	0	0	0.36	0	4
MM	90	0	0	0.32	0.06	50
DCP	90	0	0	0.24	0.16	28
Salt	90	0	0	0	0	5

Step-3 (fixing the constraints): To obtain the least cost feed we have some constraints for each nutrient, and it is unique for each animal. The minimum and maximum level of crude protein (CP 9.82–11%), total digestible nutrient (TDN 46.73–51%), calcium (0.38–0.8%), phosphorus (0.23–0.5%), roughage (40–80%) and concentrates (20–70%) was calculated on total dry matter intake for each type of cattle. The calculated constraints for each animal are as follows:

Constraints for Cattle 1:

1. $\sum_{i=1}^{17} DMI_i = 16.75$ kg
2. 1.644 kg $\leq \sum_{i=1}^{13} CP_i \leq 1.8425$ kg
3. 7.83 kg $\leq \sum_{i=1}^{13} TDN_i \leq 8.5425$ kg
4. 0.065 kg $\leq \sum_{i=1}^{17} Ca_i \leq 0.134$ kg
5. 0.04 kg $\leq \sum_{i=1}^{17} P_i \leq 0.08375$ kg
6. 6.7 kg $\leq \sum_{i=1}^{5} \text{Roughages}_i \leq 13.4$ kg
7. 3.35 kg $\leq \sum_{i=6}^{17} \text{Concentrates}_i \leq 11.725$ kg

Constraints for Cattle 2:

1. $\sum_{i=1}^{17} DMI_i = 16.89$ kg
2. 1.691 kg $\leq \sum_{i=1}^{13} CP_i \leq 1.8579$ kg

3. $7.793 \text{ kg} \leq \sum_{i=1}^{13} TDN_i \leq 8.6139 \text{ kg}$
4. $0.065 \text{ kg} \leq \sum_{i=1}^{17} Ca \leq 0.13512 \text{ kg}$
5. $0.04 \text{ kg} \leq \sum_{i=1}^{17} P_i \leq 0.08445 \text{ kg}$
6. $6.756 \text{ kg} \leq \sum_{i=1}^{5} \text{Roughages}_i \leq 13.512 \text{ kg}$
7. $3.378 \text{ kg} \leq \sum_{i=6}^{17} \text{Concentrates}_i \leq 11.823 \text{ kg}$

Constraints for Cattle 3:

1. $\sum_{i=1}^{17} DMI_i = 17.03 \text{ kg}$
2. $1.738 \text{ kg} \leq \sum_{i=1}^{13} CP_i \leq 1.8733 \text{ kg}$
3. $8.03 \text{kg} \leq \sum_{i=1}^{13} TDN_i \leq 8.6853 \text{ kg}$
4. $0.065 \text{ kg} \leq \sum_{i=1}^{17} Ca_i \leq 0.13624 \text{ kg}$
5. $0.04 \text{ kg} \leq \sum_{i=1}^{17} P_i \leq 0.08515 \text{ kg}$
6. $6.812 \text{ kg} \leq \sum_{i=1}^{5} \text{Roughages}_i \leq 13.624 \text{ kg}$
7. $3.406 \text{ kg} \leq \sum_{i=6}^{17} \text{Concentrates}_i \leq 11.921 \text{ kg}$

Step-4 (finding results): In this step, we find the least cost of "feedstuffs" after fulfilling constraints assigned by solving the linear programming model with various mathematical tools and then translating the obtained results as a recommendation to the farmers. The schematic diagram of the methodology followed is shown in Figure 5.1.

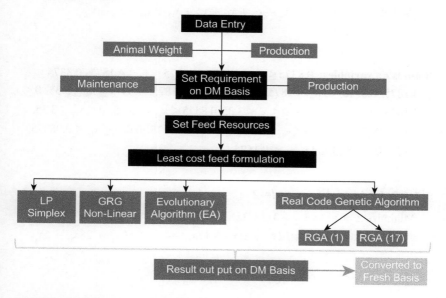

FIGURE 5.1 Schematic Diagram Representing Methodology Followed for Least Cost Feed Formulation of Dairy Cattle; Kuntal, AJAVA, 2016.

5.1.1.1 LP Model for Cattle-1

$$\text{Minimize } Z = 5x_1 + 3x_2 + 3x_3 + 3x_4 + 3x_5 + 17x_6 + 38x_7 + 23x_8$$
$$+ 23x_9 + 17x_{10} + 12x_{11} + 21x_{12} + 17x_{13} + 4x_{14}$$
$$+ 50x_{15} + 28x_{16} + 5x_{17}$$

Subjected to:

1. $x_1 + x_2 + x_3 + x_4 + x_5 + x_6 + x_7 + x_8 + x_9 + x_{10} + x_{11} + x_{12} + x_{13} + x_{14}$
   $+ x_{15} + x_{16} + x_{17} = 16.75$

2. $1.644 \leq 0.0513x_1 + 0.08x_2 + 0.08x_3 + 0.07x_4 + 0.06x_5 + 0.081x_6 + 0.42x_7$
   $+ 0.22x_8 + 0.32x_9 + 0.12x_{10} + 0.17x_{11} + 0.16x_{12} + 0.22x_{13} \leq 1.8425$

3. $7.83 \leq 0.4x_1 + 0.52x_2 + 0.6x_3 + 0.5x_4 + 0.42x_5 + 0.792x_6 + 0.7x_7 + 0.7x_8$
   $+ 0.7x_9 + 0.7x_{10} + 0.6x_{11} + 1.1x_{12} + 0.7x_{13} \leq 8.5425$

4. $0.065 \leq 0.0018x_1 + 0.00144x_2 + 0.0053x_3 + 0.0012x_4 + 0.0015x_5$
   $+ 0.00018x_6 + 0.00018x_7 + 0.00036x_8 + 0.00036x_9 + 0.01067x_{10}$
   $+ 0.000108x_{11} + 0.003x_{12} + 0.005x_{13} + 0.36x_{14} + 0.32x_{15}$
   $+ 0.24x_{16} \leq 0.134$

5. $0.04 \leq 0.0008x_1 + 0.0009x_2 + 0.0014x_3 + 0.0009x_4 + 0.0009x_5 + 0.0027x_6$
   $+ 0.00225x_7 + 0.009x_8 + 0.009x_9 + 0.00093x_{10} + 0.00234x_{11} + 0.0062x_{12}$
   $+ 0.0045x_{13} + 0.06x_{15} + 0.16x_{16} \leq 0.08375$

6. $6.7 \leq x_1 + x_2 + x_3 + x_4 + x_5 \leq 13.4$

7. $3.35 \leq x_6 + x_7 + x_8 + x_9 + x_{10} + x_{11} + x_{12} + x_{13} + x_{14} + x_{15} + x_{16}$
   $+ x_{17} \leq 11.725$

Bounds on variables: $0.8375 \leq x_1 \leq 4.1875$, $0.8375 \leq x_2 \leq 4.1875$, $0.8375 \leq x_3$ ≤ 4.1875, $0.8375 \leq x_4 \leq 4.1875$, $0.8375 \leq x_5 \leq 4.1875$, $0.8375 \leq x_6 \leq 3.35$, $0 \leq x_7$ ≤ 4.1875, $0 \leq x_8 \leq 4.1875$, $0 \leq x_9 \leq 3.35$, $0.8375 \leq x_{10} \leq 1.675$, $0 \leq x_{11} \leq 3.35$, $0 \leq x_{12} \leq 0.8375$, $0.8375 \leq x_{13} \leq 3.35$, $0 \leq x_{14} \leq 0.1675$, $0.067 \leq x_{15} \leq 0.08375$, $0 \leq x_{16} \leq 0.0335$, $0.134 \leq x_{17} \leq 0.1675$

5.1.1.2 LP Model for Cattle-2

$$\text{Minimize } Z = 5x_1 + 3x_2 + 3x_3 + 3x_4 + 3x_5 + 17x_6 + 38x_7 + 23x_8 + 23x_9$$
$$+ 17x_{10} + 12x_{11} + 21x_{12} + 17x_{13} + 4x_{14} + 50x_{15} + 28x_{16} + 5x_{17}$$

Subjected to:

1. $x_1 + x_2 + x_3 + x_4 + x_5 + x_6 + x_7 + x_8 + x_9 + x_{10} + x_{11} + x_{12} + x_{13} + x_{14} + x_{15}$
   $+ x_{16} + x_{17} = 16.89$

2. $1.691 \leq 0.0513x_1 + 0.08x_2 + 0.08x_3 + 0.07x_4 + 0.06x_5 + 0.081x_6 + 0.42x_7$
   $+ 0.22x_8 + 0.32x_9 + 0.12x_{10} + 0.17x_{11} + 0.16x_{12} + 0.22x_{13} \leq 1.8579$

3. $7.93 \leq 0.4x_1 + 0.52x_2 + 0.6x_3 + 0.5x_4 + 0.42x_5 + 0.792x_6 + 0.7x_7 + 0.7x_8$
   $+ 0.7x_9 + 0.7x_{10} + 0.6x_{11} + 1.1x_{12} + 0.7x_{13} \leq 8.6139$

4. $0.065 \leq 0.0018x_1 + 0.00144x_2 + 0.0053x_3 + 0.0012x_4 + 0.0015x_5$
   $+ 0.00018x_6 + 0.00018x_7 + 0.00036x_8 + 0.00036x_9 + 0.01067x_{10}$
   $+ 0.000108x_{11} + 0.003x_{12} + 0.005x_{13} + 0.36x_{14} + 0.32x_{15} + 0.24x_{16}$
   ≤ 0.13512

5. $0.04 \leq 0.0008x_1 + 0.0009x_2 + 0.0014x_3 + 0.0009x_4 + 0.0009x_5 + 0.0027x_6$
   $+ 0.00225x_7 + 0.009x_8 + 0.009x_9 + 0.00093x_{10} + 0.00234x_{11} + 0.0062x_{12}$
   $+ 0.0045x_{13} + 0.06x_{15} + 0.16x_{16} \leq 0.08445$

6. $6.756 \leq x_1 + x_2 + x_3 + x_4 + x_5 \leq 13.512$

7. $3.378 \leq x_6 + x_7 + x_8 + x_9 + x_{10} + x_{11} + x_{12} + x_{13} + x_{14} + x_{15} + x_{16}$
   $+ x_{17} \leq 11.823$

Bounds on variables: $0.8445 \leq x_1 \leq 4.2225$, $0.8445 \leq x_2 \leq 4.2225$, $0.8445 \leq x_3$ ≤ 4.2225, $0.8445 \leq x_4 \leq 4.2225$, $0.8445 \leq x_5 \leq 4.2225$, $0.8445 \leq x_6 \leq 3.378$, $0 \leq x_7 \leq 4.2225$, $0 \leq x_8 \leq 4.2225$, $0 \leq x_9 \leq 3.378$, $0.8445 \leq x_{10} \leq 1.689$, $0 \leq x_{11}$ ≤ 3.378, $0 \leq x_{12} \leq 0.8445$, $0.8445 \leq x_{13} \leq 3.378$, $0 \leq x_{14} \leq 0.1689$, $0.06756 \leq x_{15}$ ≤ 0.8445, $0 \leq x_{16} \leq 0.03378$, $0.13512 \leq x_{17} \leq 0.1689$

5.1.1.3 LP Model for Cattle-3

Minimize $Z = 5x_1 + 3x_2 + 3x_3 + 3x_4 + 3x_5 + 17x_6 + 38x_7 + 23x_8 + 23x_9$
$+ 17x_{10} + 12x_{11} + 21x_{12} + 17x_{13} + 4x_{14} + 50x_{15} + 28x_{16} + 5x_{17}$

Subjected to:

1. $x_1 + x_2 + x_3 + x_4 + x_5 + x_6 + x_7 + x_8 + x_9 + x_{10} + x_{11} + x_{12} + x_{13} + x_{14} + x_{15}$
   $+ x_{16} + x_{17} = 17.03$

2. $1.738 \leq 0.0513x_1 + 0.08x_2 + 0.08x_3 + 0.07x_4 + 0.06x_5 + 0.081x_6 + 0.42x_7$
   $+ 0.22x_8 + 0.32x_9 + 0.12x_{10} + 0.17x_{11} + 0.16x_{12} + 0.22x_{13} \leq 1.8733$

3. $8.03 \leq 0.4x_1 + 0.52x_2 + 0.6x_3 + 0.5x_4 + 0.42x_5 + 0.792x_6 + 0.7x_7 + 0.7x_8$
   $+ 0.7x_9 + 0.7x_{10} + 0.6x_{11} + 1.1x_{12} + 0.7x_{13} \leq 8.6853$

4. $0.065 \leq 0.0018x_1 + 0.00144x_2 + 0.0053x_3 + 0.0012x_4 + 0.0015x_5$
   $+ 0.00018x_6 + 0.00018x_7 + 0.00036x_8 + 0.00036x_9 + 0.01067x_{10}$
   $+ 0.000108x_{11} + 0.003x_{12} + 0.005x_{13} + 0.36x_{14} + 0.32x_{15} + 0.24x_{16}$
   ≤ 0.13624

5. $0.04 \leq 0.0008x_1 + 0.0009x_2 + 0.0014x_3 + 0.0009x_4 + 0.0009x_5 + 0.0027x_6$
   $+ 0.00225x_7 + 0.009x_8 + 0.009x_9 + 0.00093x_{10} + 0.00234x_{11} + 0.0062x_{12}$
   $+ 0.0045x_{13} + 0.06x_{15} + 0.16x_{16} \leq 0.08515$

6. $6.812 \leq x_1 + x_2 + x_3 + x_4 + x_5 \leq 13.624$

7. $3.406 \leq x_6 + x_7 + x_8 + x_9 + x_{10} + x_{11} + x_{12} + x_{13} + x_{14} + x_{15} + x_{16}$
   $+ x_{17} \leq 11.921$

Bounds on variables: $0.8515 \leq x_1 \leq 4.2575$, $0.8515 \leq x_2 \leq 4.2225$, $0.8515 \leq x_3 \leq 4.2225$, $0.8515 \leq x_4 \leq 4.2225$, $0.8515 \leq x_5 \leq 4.2225$, $0.8515 \leq x_6 \leq 3.406$, $0 \leq x_7 \leq 4.2575$, $0 \leq x_8 \leq 4.2575$, $0 \leq x_9 \leq 3.406$, $0.8515 \leq x_{10} \leq 1.703$, $0 \leq x_{11} \leq 3.406$, $0 \leq x_{12} \leq 0.8515$, $0.8515 \leq x_{13} \leq 3.406$, $0 \leq x_{14} \leq 0.1703$, $0.06812 \leq x_{15} \leq 0.08515$, $0 \leq x_{16} \leq 0.03406$, $0.13624 \leq x_{17} \leq 0.1703$

5.2 Implementation

As suggested by Ghosh et al., (2014), we have explored the possibility of using various techniques including genetic algorithm (GA) to solve the feed formulation problem (refer to Chapter 4). The success of GA is in its evolution process. More recently, real coded genetic algorithm (RGA) has been used in numerical optimization (Herrera et al., 1995; Ono et al., 2003), and most of the optimization is done in real space (continuous space). However, constraints are rigid; the use of RGA overcomes the low resolution of solution weakness of binary coded GA (Baron et al., 2002; Achiche et al., 2002). The outline of RGA is as follows:

Step-1: Genetic algorithm starts with first creating the initial population randomly. In MATLAB 2013, if we set the population size, then the initial population generated by the algorithm is same as population size by default, so to solve our linear programming problem we have generated a 500-population size.

Step-2: Sequence of new population and next generation: This creates a sequence of new population using RGA operators, namely crossover, mutation and selection. At every step of RGA, the current population is used to form new offspring that create the next generation. The current population selected is called parents and the generated new population is called offspring. RGA selects the best fit population as parents to generate new offspring, which is done by selection operator. RGA provides three types of offspring for the next generation, namely crossover offspring, mutation offspring and elite offspring. Crossover offspring are created by the crossover operator, which shows how GA combines two parents to undergo crossover for creating crossover children. In our case, we have used a heuristic crossover method to generate the children, because it moves from worst parent to past best parent. We have used the default ratio 1.2, where this ratio indicates how far offspring is from the better parent. If P_1 and P_2 are two parents, where P_1 is having a better fitness value, then child = P_2 + Ratio $(P_1 - P_2)$. Mutation offspring can be created by randomly changing individuals in the population. It is an important operator to maintain diversity and search broader spaces. In our study we have used adaptive feasible mutation because it performs better on linear constraints. It randomly generates directions that are adaptive with respect to its previous generation. This method chooses the direction and step length that satisfies linear constraints. Elite offspring are created based on positive integer values after crossover or mutation operators, which specify how many best fit offspring are guaranteed to survive in each generation. We have kept the elite count at 2, and it is a good operator for the convergence point of view; keeping a high value of elite count does not guarantee good convergence, as we need some worst fit solution every generation as well. We used a tournament selection procedure, which selects parent by selecting tournament size at random and then selecting best fit parents. We kept default tournament size at 4. We also used the initial penalty as 10 and penalty factor as 100, where initial penalty specifies the initial penalty used for nonlinear constraint and the penalty will increase the penalty parameter whenever there are constraint violations or whenever the problem is not providing accuracy. Generally, this option of RGA is used for nonlinear constraints, but as we have rigid constraints and bounds, we have used penalty factors as an option to optimize the problem (Kuntal et al., 2016, 2018).

Step-3: Stopping criteria of the algorithm: We have used generation as a stopping criterion, where once the maximum generation is reached, the algorithm stops and the exit flag gives the reason why the algorithm has stopped.

5.2.1 Results and Discussions

The results obtained by various techniques, viz. LP simplex, GRG nonlinear, evolutionary algorithm (EA) and real coded genetic algorithm (RGA), with seeding the random numbers for least cost ration by LP model are presented in Tables 5.4, 5.6 and 5.8 for Cattle-1, 2 and 3 on a DM basis, respectively. LP model-1, 2

TABLE 5.4

Least Cost of Ration by Various Techniques for Cattle-1 on DM Basis

Variables	Simplex & GRG nonlinear	EA with seeding	RGA with RNG (1)	RGA with RNG (17)
x_1	3.3184369	3.46200246	3.1889	2.8845
x_2	3.1048270	1.88904534	3.0043	2.8115
x_3	0.8375	1.13120299	0.8375	0.8375
x_4	4.1875	0.87935706	1.5299	1.7039
x_5	0.8375	1.87331391	3.7707	4.0965
x_6	0.8375	1.15084533	0.8375	0.8375
x_7	0	0.14970428	0.2189	0.2203
x_8	0	0.67154322	0	0
x_9	1.5497360	0.38100715	1.2351	1.2311
x_{10}	0.8375	1.43585220	0.8375	0.8375
x_{11}	0	0.85084407	0	0
x_{12}	0	0.14824419	0	0
x_{13}	0.8375	2.11359082	0.8375	0.8375
x_{14}	0.1675	0.15013463	0.1675	0.1675
x_{15}	0.067	0.06981443	0.0837	0.0838
x_{16}	0	0.01619651	0.0335	0.0335
x_{17}	0.1675	0.16741651	0.1675	0.1675
CP	1.644	1.82458530	1.6440	1.644
TDN	8.5425000	9.18352968	8.5425	8.5425
Calcium	0.1176172	0.12612679	0.1309	0.1308
Phosphorus	0.0419254	0.04198480	0.0400	0.04
Roughage	12.285764	9.23492177	12.3313	12.3339
Concentrate	4.4642360	7.30519339	4.4187	4.4162
DMI	16.75	16.5401151	16.7500	16.7501
Least cost	126.708094	163.136196	129.4403	128.8009

TABLE 5.5

Least Cost of Ration by Various Techniques for Cattle-1 on As Fresh Basis (LP Model)

Variables	Simplex & GRG nonlinear	RGA without seeding RNG	RGA with RNG (1)	Real coded GA with RNG (17)
x_1	3.687152	3.084888889	3.543222222	3.205
x_2	12.41931	10.4672	12.0172	11.246
x_3	3.35	3.35	3.35	3.35
x_4	4.652778	2.126555556	1.699888889	1.893222222
x_5	0.930556	4.652777778	4.189666667	4.551666667
x_6	0.930556	0.930555556	0.930555556	0.930555556
x_7	0	0.249	0.243222222	0.244777778
x_8	0	0	0	0
x_9	1.721929	1.365666667	1.372333333	1.367888889

Variables	Simplex & GRG nonlinear	RGA without seeding RNG	RGA with RNG (1)	Real coded GA with RNG (17)
x_{10}	0.930556	0.930555556	0.930555556	0.930555556
x_{11}	0	0	0	0
x_{12}	0	0	0	0
x_{13}	0.930556	0.930555556	0.930555556	0.930555556
x_{14}	0.17268	0.172680412	0.172680412	0.172680412
x_{15}	0.074444	0.093111111	0.093	0.093111111
x_{16}	0	0.037222222	0.037222222	0.037222222
x_{17}	0.186111	0.186111111	0.186111111	0.186111111
TMR as fresh basis (in kg)	29.98663	28.57688041	29.69621375	29.13934708
Least cost in Rs on as fresh basis	174.8999	172.8637661	177.0643216	174.688055
Least cost (Rs/kg)	5.832596	6.049078	5.962522	5.99492

TABLE 5.6

Least Cost of Ration by Various Techniques for Cattle-2 on DM Basis (LP Model)

Variables	Simplex & GRG nonlinear	EA with seeding	RGA With RNG (1)	RGA With RNG (17)
x_1	3.5268827	3.4909386	3.4237	4.2225
x_2	2.7694622	1.9048344	2.3255	0.8445
x_3	0.8445	1.1406578	0.8445	0.8445
x_4	0.8445	0.8867069	1.4873	3.8991
x_5	4.2225	1.8889715	3.8958	2.4448
x_6	0.8444	1.1604643	0.8445	0.8445
x_7	0	0.1509555	0.3213	0.4701
x_8	0	0.6771561	0.0563	0.0933
x_9	1.7280454	0.3841917	1.0548	1.0817
x_{10}	0.8444	1.4478534	0.8445	0.8445
x_{11}	0	0.8579556	0.4912	0
x_{12}	0	0.1494833	0.0000	0
x_{13}	0.8445	2.1312567	0.8445	0.8445
x_{14}	0.1689	0.1513895	0.1689	0.1689
x_{15}	0.06756	0.070398	0.0844	0.0844
x_{16}	0.0154497	0.0163319	0.0338	0.0338
x_{17}	0.1689	0.1688158	0.1689	0.1689
CP	1.691	1.8398356	1.6910	1.691
TDN	8.6139	9.2602875	8.6139	8.6139
Calcium	0.1222969	0.127181	0.1319	0.1315
Phosphorus	0.04	0.0423357	0.0401	0.04
Roughage	12.207845	9.3121092	11.9768	12.2554
Concentrate	4.6821551	7.3662517	4.9131	4.6346
DMI	16.89	16.678361	16.8899	16.89
Least cost	131.81914	164.49972	136.1944	139.856

TABLE 5.7

Least Cost of Ration by Various Techniques for Cattle-2 on As Fresh Basis (LP Model)

Variables	Simplex & GRG nonlinear	RGA without seeding RNG	RGA with RNG (1)	RGA with RNG (17)
x_1	3.919248	3.284889	3.804111	4.691667
x_2	11.07516	10.1896	9.302	3.378
x_3	3.378	3.378	3.378	3.378
x_4	0.938333	1.974222	1.652556	4.332333
x_5	4.691667	4.691667	4.328667	2.716444
x_6	0.938333	0.938333	0.938333	0.938333
x_7	0	0.420222	0.357	0.522333
x_8	0	0	0.062556	0.103667
x_9	1.920089	1.305222	1.172	1.201889
x_{10}	0.938333	0.938333	0.938333	0.938333
x_{11}	0	0	0.545778	0
x_{12}	0	0	0	0
x_{13}	0.938333	0.938333	0.938333	0.938333
x_{14}	0.174124	0.174124	0.174124	0.174124
x_{15}	0.075067	0.093889	0.093778	0.093778
x_{16}	0.017163	0.037556	0.037556	0.037556
x_{17}	0.187667	0.187667	0.187667	0.187667
TMR on as fresh basis in kg)	29.19152	28.55206	27.91079	23.63246
Least cost in Rs on as fresh basis	177.7315	178.3493	178.7446	169.9794
Least cost (Rs/kg)	6.088463	6.24646	6.40414	7.192624

TABLE 5.8

Least Cost of Ration by Various Techniques for Cattle-3 on DM Basis (LP Model)

Variables	Simplex & GRG nonlinear	EA with seeding	RGA with RNG (1)	RGA with RNG (17)
x_1	3.85658052	3.5198747	3.1263	3.5056
x_2	2.33299069	1.9206234	2.323	2.4336
x_3	0.8514	1.1501126	0.8515	0.8515
x_4	0.8515	0.8940567	1.82	1.7554
x_5	4.2575	1.9046290	4.2393	3.8079
x_6	0.8514	1.1700833	0.8515	0.8515
x_7	0	0.1522068	0.5362	0.5378
x_8	0	0.6827690	0	0
x_9	1.91220552	0.3873762	1.1195	1.1239
x_{10}	0.8514	1.4598545	0.8515	0.8515
x_{11}	0	0.8650671	0	0
x_{12}	0	0.1507223	0	0

Variables	Simplex & GRG nonlinear	EA with seeding	RGA with RNG (1)	RGA with RNG (17)
x_{13}	0.8515	2.1489224	0.8515	0.8515
x_{14}	0.17025892	0.1526443	0.1703	0.1703
x_{15}	0.06812	0.0709814	0.0851	0.0852
x_{16}	0.00503889	0.0164672	0.0341	0.0341
x_{17}	0.1703	0.1702151	0.1703	0.1703
CP	1.73800000	1.8550858	1.7380	1.738
TDN	8.68530003	9.3370454	8.6854	8.6853
Calcium	0.12070605	0.1282351	0.1327	0.1329
Phosphorus	0.04	0.0426866	0.0400	0.04
Roughage	12.1499712	9.3892965	12.3601	12.354
Concentrate	4.88012333	7.4273100	4.6700	4.676
DMI	17.0300945	16.816606	17.0301	17.03
Least cost	136.644426	165.86324	139.6257	140.5297

TABLE 5.9

Least Cost of Ration by Various Techniques for Cattle-3 on As Fresh Basis

Variables	Simplex & GRG nonlinear	RGA without seeding RNG	RGA with RNG (1)	RGA with RNG (17)
x_1	4.285569	3.44955555	3.4736666	3.895111
x_2	9.327939	8.3764	9.292	9.7344
x_3	3.406	3.406	3.406	3.406
x_4	0.946111	2.31666666	2.0222222	1.9504444
x_5	4.730556	4.68933333	4.7103333	4.231
x_6	0.946111	0.94611111	0.9461111	0.946111111
x_7	0	0.60211111	0.5957777	0.597555556
x_8	0	0	0	0
x_9	2.124722	1.24244444	1.2438888	1.248777778
x_{10}	0.946111	0.94611111	0.9461111	0.946111111
x_{11}	0	0	0	0
x_{12}	0	0	0	0
x_{13}	0.946111	0.94611111	0.9461111	0.946111111
x_{14}	0.175567	0.17556701	0.1755670	0.17556701
x_{15}	0.075689	0.09466666	0.0945555	0.094666667
x_{16}	0.005592	0.03788888	0.0378888	0.037888889
x_{17}	0.189222	0.18922222	0.1892222	0.189222222
TMR as fresh basis (in kg)	28.1053	27.4181892	28.079455	28.39896701
Least cost in Rs on as fresh basis	179.3693	180.763690	182.59771	184.5643569
Least cost (Rs/kg)	6.382045	6.592838	6.502894	6.498981

TABLE 5.10

Net Profit Per Cattle in INR to Farmers for 10 Litres of Milk on As Fresh Basis Each Day

Level	Milk rate in dairy (INR)	Net profit by simplex LP & GRG nonlinear	Net profit by RGA without seeding	Net profit by RGA with RNG (1)	Net profit by RGA with RNG (17)
Cattle-1	22.6	51.1001	53.13623	48.93568	51.311945
Cattle-2	22.6	48.2685	47.6507	47.2554	56.0206
Cattle-3	22.6	46.6307	45.23631	43.40229	41.4356431
Mean ± S. E		48.67±1.31	48.67±2.34	46.53±1.64	49.59±4.30
P value	0.868 NS				

NS–Non-significance: P > 0.05. No significance difference exists between methods.

and 3 for each type of cattle have 17 variables, which are too complex for finding an optimal solution graphically; hence, we used the LP simplex method, which provides an iterative algorithm to locate the corner points systematically until we get an optimal solution. A GRG nonlinear algorithm with forward differencing deals with problems involving decision variables and nonlinear constraints. Forward differencing uses a single point that is slightly different from current value to find the derivative; hence, while solving LP models in Excel Solver, it will not compute derivatives again and again, and it continues to estimate the solution along the straight line instead of recalculating the changing gradients. When GRG finds a solution, this means that solver has found a valley for minimizing the objective function after satisfying the Karush-Kuhn-Tucker (KKT) conditions for local optimality, and there is no other possible solution for decision variables (feedstuffs) near to current values. The evolutionary algorithm (EA) technique is also used to solve LP model by seeding the random number generator. In the present study, the EA method with seeding technique could not find a lower least cost than the other three methods because costlier nutrients like the crude protein level in final feed was higher (1.82 kg) in EA than other methods (1.644 kg). Similarly, the TDN content is higher in the EA method than other methods. These could be the reason for higher costs in EA (INR 163.14) than the other methods (GRG-126.71; LP- 126.71: RGA seeding 1–129.44 and RGA seeding 17–128.8). It is evident that the EA method had a not so accurate least cost feed formulation method because it uses only mutation as a parameter to improve the diversity of the population in every generation. The EA method is heuristic in nature and uses only mutation as a parameter to improve the diversity of the problem; hence, while solving the problem the constraints are not satisfied properly and almost all the constraints are violated. If we do not seed the random number, then we get the wide ranges of solutions in every run most of the time, but unfortunately in this study we have not achieved the optimal solution using EA in MS Excel Solver due to the rigidity of the constraints. The RGA with seeding technique is applied to overcome the limitation of EA. RGA is also a heuristic technique which works on the principle of survival of best fit and tournament selection. Adaptive feasibility mutation and heuristic crossover is used along with elitism to solve the LP model for Cattle-1, 2 and 3. Though the seeding technique gives a near optimal answer, we prefer to provide a wide ranges of solutions to farmers in which the values of feedstuffs changes in every run where all the constraints will satisfy. As a farmer needs the total mixed ration to feed the cattle on an "as fresh basis", we have converted the least cost and total mixed ration obtained by all techniques to as fresh basis, and the results are given in Tables 5.5, 5.7 and 5.9. As per the fitment in Table 5.4, each animal of the Cattle-1 category requires about 16.75 kg of dry matter from various feed ingredients which should contain 1644 g of protein, 8542 g of TDN, 117.6 g of calcium and 42 g of phosphorus, and these nutrients can be met from 12.29 kg of roughages and 4.464 kg of concentrate on dry matter. The corresponding total mixed ration (TMR) cost on dry matter basis is Rs 126.70, that is, Rs 7.56 per kg, because fresh basis is a feed nutrient content with moisture included. After converting to as fresh basis, the feedstuff requirement for Cattle-1 is approximately 30 kg/day, amounting to Rs 5.83/kg using the GRG nonlinear and simplex LP technique. When RGA was used to try to achieve the expected nutrient requirement without seeding and with seeding (RGA1 and RGA17), the least cost ration obtained was Rs 6.05/kg, Rs 5.96/kg and Rs 5.99/kg, respectively. The detailed analysis of the ration showed (in Tables 5.3 and 5.4) that it exactly met the requirement of dry matter, TDN, CP, calcium and phosphorus, and roughage: the concentrate was also well within the permissible range. Similar analysis has been done for Cattle-2 (see Tables 5.6 and 5.7), where the least cost ration obtained by various techniques for as fresh basis is Rs 6.08, Rs 6.25, Rs 6.40 and Rs 7.20 per kg by LP simplex, GRG nonlinear, RGA1 and RGA17, respectively. For Cattle-3 (see Tables 5.8 and 5.9), the TMR cost for as fresh basis turns out to be Rs 6.38, Rs 6.59, Rs 6.50 and Rs 6.50 per kg, respectively. Table 5.9 shows the net profit that farmers can make per cattle in Indian rupees for 10 litres of milk each day on an as fresh basis by all techniques. A one-way ANOVA test at 5% level of significance has been performed for the "Null hypothesis: there is no significant difference between techniques", the test reveals that since the P value is greater than 0.05, there is no significance difference between the techniques. Hence, it is proved that the real parameters-based genetic algorithm (www.scialert.net) can be effectively used for low-cost diet formulation of dairy cattle.

5.2.2 Conclusion

This study addresses the use of RGA as a tool to provide good quality feed mix to dairy cattle for better health and milk production. All the techniques – viz. LP simplex, GRG nonlinear, evolutionary algorithm (EA) and real coded genetic algorithm (RGA) with seeding the random numbers – for least cost ration are performing equally. Hence, it is concluded that RGA (www.scialert.net) will give low-cost diet formulation for dairy cattle. However, the fixing of constrains and use of code for making software is also be considered while choosing the techniques for making least cost feed formulation. Further detailed research with various species of animals and with different physiological needs may require to fine-tune the techniques for farmer use. We also tried to cut down cost of TMR without any shortage of nutrients in the diet.

5.3 A Goal Programming Approach to Ration Formulation Problem for Indian Dairy Cows

Due to the limitation of feedstuffs in the Mandya district of Karnataka, small dairy farmers faced many problems to feed a balanced, least cost diet to dairy cattle. From earlier research it was clear that the productivity of cattle maintained by different dairy farmers was lower, and this is mainly due to limited resources for feeding and small farmers not having proper knowledge or resources to provide a low-cost balanced ration to cattle. Therefore, there is a need to focus on minimizing the diet cost by upgrading scientific dairy farming practices. Several techniques are in use for animal diet formulation, but a successful application of a soft computing technique to improve the quality of the solution is always preferred, as the rigidity of the functions in a linear programming problem (LPP) can be easily handled. Hence, to meet the nutrient requirement, a primitive goal programming (GP) model for three categories of dairy cattle weighing 500 kg each and yielding 10 litres of milk with 4% fat content during the seventh, eighth and ninth month of pregnancy has been formulated by dividing the goals into a set of priorities. In our earlier work (Kuntal et al., 2016), LP models for three categories of dairy cattle has been formulated and solved by the simplex method, GRG nonlinear method, EA method and real coded genetic method (RGA). In the present work, a GP model has been developed by dividing each goal into a set of priorities for all three categories of animal, as there are two high priority objectives – least cost and dry matter intake – to be achieved if possible. This GP model is solved by a real coded genetic algorithm with hybrid function (RHGA), which shows that five goals are overachieved, while one goal is fully achieved and one is underachieved for Cattle-1 and 2. It can be concluded that the real parameter-based hybrid genetic algorithm can also find a low-cost diet plan without violating the nutrient requirements (www.scialert.net).

India has the largest livestock population in world. Livestock is one of the country's most important economic activities, especially in the rural areas of country, providing income for most of the family. In dairy farming, feeding costs account for about 70% of the total operation cost. The dairying programme has attained considerable importance in various Five-Year Plans, and the states and the Centre have taken up several schemes/projects for the development of this sector, but a different diet plan is needed for different categories of dairy cows: calculating the low-cost balanced diet requires an understanding of the nutrient requirements of dairy cows in different conditions. As per the 19th livestock census report, the population of cows has increased by 6.52% over the previous census report (2007), and the total number of cows estimated in 2012 was 122.9 million. The total number of milking animals in India is 116.77 million, of which 12% of the contribution is from cattle (Babic et al., 2011). Also, as per the Basic

Animal Husbandry and Fisheries Statistics 2017, the per capita availability of average milk in Karnataka was 291 grams per day during 2016–17, which is less than the 12 top milk-producing states in India such as Uttar Pradesh. Karnataka has only a 4% share in milk production for the year 2016–17. From 2012 to 2016, the cattle population increased from 1142.62 to 1370.69 (in thousands), with an estimated milk production of 5718.22 to 6562.15 (in thousands of kg) in which the average yield per in-milk animal of nondescript/indigenous cows from 2012–13 to 2016–17 in Karnataka was 2.32–2.43 kg/day. Area under fodder crops increased from 35000 hectares to 36000 hectares in 2006–07, and permanent pastures and other grazing lands decreased from 930000 hectares to 906000 hectares from 2006–07 to 2013–14 (Basic Animal Husbandry & Fisheries Statistics, 2017). According to past surveys, it was clear that farmers are not feeding dairy cattle properly due to high feed cost and unavailability of proper feedstuffs (Garg, 2012). Therefore, it is necessary to supply a least cost balanced diet to dairy cattle, especially during pregnancy and the milking period. Since 1991 many researchers have studied feeding practices in which small farmers have limited resources for feeding practices (Leng, 1991: 82). The livestock industry plays an important role in the development of the Indian economy, as the livestock sector in agriculture GDP increased from 13.88% to 29.20% from 1990 to 2013. The livestock sector also amounts to 4% of the national GDP (Department of Animal Husbandry, Annual Report, 2016–17; Angadi et al., 2016). Hence, when considering the economic importance and difficulties of Indian farmers, an improvement in feeding practice is required which results in a least cost feed plan for dairy cows at different hypothetical conditions. Linear programming (LP) is one of the commonly utilized strategies pursued by many economical and non-economical diet formulation programs, but Rehman and Romero described the limitation of LP while formulating a low-cost diet plan. The inference in the linear programming model restricts the constraints (to be fixed in RHS) and objective functions to a single objective, which implies an application of the goal programming model which consists of constraints and sets of goals, which are sometimes prioritized (Gupta et al., 2013b: 414–422). The main reason to apply a GP model is to satisfy all the constraints in terms of goals. Basically, goals can be satisfied completely or partially, or sometimes goals cannot be met. This problem where goals cannot be met can be handled by adding +*ve* and −*ve* deviational variables which are defined for each goal individually. After all, the objective function of a weighted goal programming model optimizes the sum of the total deviation from set goals where the outcome may lead to a compromise solution between contradictory goals (Gupta et al., 2013b: 414–422). Zoran Babic et al. applied a goal programming method to determine an optimal blend of ingredients for livestock feed in which a GP-based model turns out to be a useful method in deciding the optimal livestock diet formulation (Babic, 2011). Evolutionary algorithms (EAs) consist of genetic algorithms (GAs), genetic programming and their hybrid functions (Rehman [Ph.D. thesis] 2014), and an EA highly depends upon its operators (Koda, 2012: 1–16). Furuya et al. in 1997 used genetic algorithms in which the ratio of ingredients has evolved. Sahman et al. used a GA to find a least cost diet for livestock, which results in a good solution with few constraints

(Şahman et al., 2009: 965–974). Shilpa Jain et al. did the comparative analysis of a real and binary coded genetic algorithm on a fuzzy time series prediction. The authors concluded that the real coded GA runs much faster than a binary coded GA (Shilpa et al., 2013: 299–304). In a previous case study, an LP model of dairy cows weighing 500 kg which are pregnant at three different months (seventh, eighth and ninth months) was formulated and solved using LP simplex, GRG nonlinear, EA and different parameters of a real coded genetic algorithm based on primary data. This study resulted in "no significance difference between techniques" ($p > 0.05$) and concluded that RGA can be used to formulate the least cost diet. In this case study we have extended the work to formulate the goal programming model of dairy cows, which are pregnant at third trimester, that is, in the seventh, eighth and ninth month, which required a balanced diet to maintain health and to produce milk with 4% fat (Kuntal et al., 2016: 594–607). This GP model is solved using a real coded hybrid genetic algorithm.

5.3.1 Goal Programming Approach

In accord with the nutritionist, it was decided to try the linear model developed by (Kuntal et al., 2016) by formulating it into goal programming models. In earlier work, a linear model for Cattle-1, Cattle-2 and Cattle-3 had been developed for cows with a body weight of 500 kg which is pregnant at third trimester that requires a balanced ration for body maintenance and 10 litres of milk production with 4% fat. Three goal programming models for these cattle was formulated by considering several goals, where all the constraints except dry matter intake (DMI) are given priority and in which least cost is highly prioritized. In earlier work, the upper and lower bounds for each constraint has been set by the decision maker as per the Indian Council of Agricultural Research–ICAR 2013 and NRC 2001 standard. In this chapter, the constraints are converted to goals; their target values on a dry matter basis to find the diet plan are:

1. The cost should be Rs 126.71/- for Cattle-1, Rs 131.82/- for Cattle-2 and Rs 136.65/- for Cattle-3.
2. Total dry matter intake (DMI) will be 16.75 kg for Cattle-1, 16.89 kg for Cattle-2 and 17.03 kg for Cattle-3.
3. Crude protein (CP) will be 1.644 kg for Cattle-1, 1.691kg for Cattle-2 and 1.738 kg for Cattle-3.
4. Total digestible nutrients (TDN) will be 8.5425 kg for Cattle-1, 8.6139 kg for Cattle-2 and 8.6853 for Cattle-3.
5. Calcium (Ca) will be 0.1176 kg for Cattle-1, 0.1223 kg for Cattle-2 and 0.1207 kg for Cattle-3.
6. Phosphorus will be 0.04193 kg for Cattle-1 and 0.04 for Cattle-2 and 3.
7. Roughage will be 12.2858 kg for Cattle-1, 12.2076 kg for Cattle-2 and 12.1495 kg for Cattle-3.

8. Concentrates will be 4.4642 kg for Cattle-1, 4.6824 kg for Cattle-2 and 4.8805 kg for Cattle-3. This forms the GP model in which seven goals (except DMI) are formulated as goal functions. It is not easy to meet all the seven goals; therefore, deviational variables are introduced. The achievement (objective) function of the GP model becomes the sum of the square root of deviation variables, which required minimization. This goal-programming model is solved by a real coded hybrid genetic algorithm.

5.3.1.1 GP Model-1

$$Min\ (Z) = \sqrt{\begin{array}{c} p_1\left(d_{\text{cost}}^{+}\right)^2 + p_2\left(d_{CP}^{-}\right)^2 + p_3\left(d_{TDN}^{-}\right)^2 + p_4\left(d_{Ca}^{-}\right)^2 + p_5\left(d_{Ph}^{-}\right)^2 \\ + p_6\left(d_{\text{Rough}}^{-}\right)^2 + p_7\left(d_{\text{Conc}}^{-}\right)^2 \end{array}}$$

Subjected to:

1. Goal 1(Minimize Least Cost): $\sum_{i=1}^{17} C_i x_i + d_{\text{cost}}^{-} - d_{\text{cost}}^{+} = 126.71$

2. Goal 2(Maximize Crude Protein): $\sum_{i=1}^{17} CP_i + d_{CP}^{-} - d_{CP}^{+} = 1.644\ \text{Kg}$

3. Goal 3(Maximize Total Digestible Nutrient): $\sum_{i=1}^{17} TDN_i + d_{TDN}^{-} - d_{TDN}^{+}$
   $$= 8.5425\ \text{Kg}$$

4. Goal 4(Maximize Calcium): $\sum_{i=1}^{17} Ca_i + d_{Ca}^{-} - d_{Ca}^{+} = 0.1176\ \text{Kg}$

5. Goal 5(Maximize Phosphorus): $\sum_{i=1}^{17} Ph_i + d_{Ph}^{-} - d_{Ph}^{+} = 0.04193\ \text{Kg}$

6. Goal 6(Maximize Roughages): $\sum_{i=1}^{5} \text{Rough}_i + d_{\text{Rough}}^{-} - d_{\text{Rough}}^{+} = 12.2858\ \text{K}$

7. Goal 7(Maximize Concentrates): $\sum_{i=6}^{17} \text{Conc}_i + d_{\text{Conc}}^{-} - d_{\text{Conc}}^{+} = 4.4642\ \text{Kg}$

8. $\sum_{i=1}^{17} x_i = 16.75\ \text{Kg}$

5.3.1.2 GP Model-2

$$Min\ (Z) = \sqrt{\begin{array}{c} p_1\left(d_{\text{cost}}^{+}\right)^2 + p_2\left(d_{CP}^{-}\right)^2 + p_3\left(d_{TDN}^{-}\right)^2 + p_4\left(d_{Ca}^{-}\right)^2 + p_5\left(d_{Ph}^{-}\right)^2 \\ + p_6\left(d_{\text{Rough}}^{-}\right)^2 + p_7\left(d_{\text{Conc}}^{-}\right)^2 \end{array}}$$

Subjected to:

1. Goal 1(Minimize Least Cost): $\sum_{i=1}^{17} C_i x_i + d_{\text{cost}}^{-} - d_{\text{cost}}^{+} = 131.8234$

2. Goal 2 (Maximize Crude Protein): $\sum_{i=1}^{17} CP_i + d_{CP}^{-} - d_{CP}^{+} = 1.691 \, \text{Kg}$

3. Goal 3 (Maximize Total Digestible Nutrient): $\sum_{i=1}^{17} TDN_i + d_{TDN}^{-} - d_{TDN}^{+}$
$$= 8.6139 \, \text{Kg}$$

4. Goal 4 (Maximize Calcium): $\sum_{i=1}^{17} Ca_i + d_{Ca}^{-} - d_{Ca}^{+} = 0.1223 \, \text{Kg}$

5. Goal 5 (Maximize Phosphorus): $\sum_{i=1}^{17} Ph_i + d_{Ph}^{-} - d_{Ph}^{+} = 0.04 \, \text{Kg}$

6. Goal 6 (Maximize Roughages): $\sum_{i=1}^{17} \text{Rough}_i + d_{\text{Rough}}^{-} - d_{\text{Rough}}^{+} = 12.2076 \, \text{Kg}$

7. Goal 7 (Maximize Concentrates): $\sum_{i=6}^{17} \text{Conc}_i + d_{\text{Conc}}^{-} - d_{\text{Conc}}^{+} = 4.6824 \, \text{Kg}$

8. $\sum_{i=1}^{17} x_i = 16.89 \, \text{Kg}$

5.3.1.3 GP Model-3

$$Min\,(Z) = \sqrt{\begin{array}{l} p_1 \left(d_{\text{cost}}^{+}\right)^2 + p_2 \left(d_{CP}^{-}\right)^2 + p_3 \left(d_{TDN}^{-}\right)^2 + p_4 \left(d_{Ca}^{-}\right)^2 + p_5 \left(d_{Ph}^{-}\right)^2 \\ + p_6 \left(d_{\text{Rough}}^{-}\right)^2 + p_7 \left(d_{\text{Conc}}^{-}\right)^2 \end{array}}$$

Subjected to:

1. Goal 1 (Minimize Least Cost): $\sum_{i=1}^{17} C_i x_i + d_{\text{cost}}^{-} - d_{\text{cost}}^{+} = 136.65$

2. Goal 2 (Maximize Crude Protein): $\sum_{i=1}^{17} CP_i + d_{CP}^{-} - d_{CP}^{+} = 1.738 \, \text{Kg}$

3. Goal 3 (Maximize Total Digestible Nutrient): $\sum_{i=1}^{17} TDN_i + d_{TDN}^{-} - d_{TDN}^{+}$
$$= 8.6853 \, \text{Kg}$$

4. Goal 4 (Maximize Calcium): $\sum_{i=1}^{17} Ca_i + d_{Ca}^{-} - d_{Ca}^{+} = 0.1207 \, \text{Kg}$

5. Goal 5 (Maximize Phosphorus): $\sum_{i=1}^{17} Ph_i + d_{Ph}^{-} - d_{Ph}^{+} = 0.04 \, \text{Kg}$

6. Goal 6 (Maximize Roughages): $\sum_{i=1}^{5} \text{Rough}_i + d_{\text{Rough}}^{-} - d_{\text{Rough}}^{+} = 12.1495 \, \text{Kg}$

7. Goal 7 (Maximize Concentrates): $\sum_{i=6}^{17} \text{Conc}_i + d_{\text{Conc}}^{-} - d_{\text{Conc}}^{+} = 4.8805 \, \text{Kg}$

8. $\sum_{i=1}^{17} x_i = 17.03 \, \text{Kg}$

where $p_i (i = 1, 2 \ldots 7)$ are positive numbers between $(0,1)$ such that $p_1 > p_2 > \ldots p_7$.

5.3.2 Real Coded Genetic Algorithm with Hybrid Function

Genetic algorithm is a search-based technique which is based on evolutionary theory. Binary coded GA represents decision variables by bits of zeros and ones, whereas GA based on real number representation is called a real coded GA (RGA). GA works on a solution space instead of a state space, where it builds new solutions based on the existing one. We first created an initial population then decided on the gene representation; we chose default population type "double vector" to represent genes. After the representation of genes, the population undergoes three major GA operators such as selection, crossover and mutation to create next generations. MATLAB provides *"gaoptimset"* to create or modify the GA option structure. In general, MATLAB fails to provide every possible method available in literature, but it provides lot of options to find the optimal solution. The selection procedure decides how individuals are selected to become parents. We used a tournament selection procedure of size 2, where individuals may be chosen more than once as a parent. Crossover combines two parents to create new offspring for the next generation. The crossover heuristic returns offspring because it moves from worst parents to past best parent, for example, if P_1 and P_2 are two parents where P_1 has better fitness then offspring $= P_2 + 1.2 \times (P_1 - P_2)$, where 1.2 is the ratio. Mutation decides how an algorithm makes small changes in the individual randomly to create new mutation offspring. Mutation is an important operator from a diversity point of view, which allows the GA to search in a broader space. We have linear constraints and bounds; hence, an adaptive feasible mutation is used which generates a direction that is flexible with regard to previous favorable or unfavorable iterations (generations). The feasible region is bounded by the equality and inequality constraints. An appropriate step length is chosen towards each direction so that linear constraints as well as bounds can be satisfied. After specifying these genetic algorithm options for linear models, the GA sometimes returns a local minimum instead of global minimum, that is, a point where the objective function value is less than the nearby points but possibly greater than the distant point in solution space. Therefore, to overcome this deficiency of GAs, we have introduced the hybrid command "fmincon" inside the GA, in which we allow the GA to find the valley that contains the global minimum and after last generation; it takes the last value of GA as the initial value of fmincon to converge quickly. In addition to that, the GA can be tested in broader space by improving the diversity of the population, and it can be done by manipulating the initial range of the population. However, we have rigid constraints and bounds, so we want to search the point in the specified lower and upper bounds only. Based on the GP model, we have 31 decision variables and seven goals (1-Equality constraint). We have to find the minimum cost of diet based on dry matter; hence, we set the number of variables to 31, from which we have developed three goal-programming models with different priorities for cows with body weight of 500 kg which are pregnant at third trimester.

5.3.3 Results

TABLE 5.11

Least Cost, Deviation, and Constraints Value Solved by Hybrid RGA for Goal
Programming Models

Variables	Feedstuffs	GP Model-1	GP Model-2	GP Model-3
x_1	Paddy straw	0	0	0
x_2	Co-4 grass	0	0	0
x_3	Maize fodder	12.2802	12.2014	12.1431
x_4	Co-FS 29 sorghum fodder	0	0	0
x_5	Ragi straw	0	0	0
x_6	Maize	0	0	0
x_7	Soya DOC	0	0	0
x_8	Copra DOC	0.0480	0	0
x_9	Cotton DOC	0.6099	0.7691	0.908
x_{10}	Wheat bran	3.7989	3.9052	3.9654
x_{11}	Gram chunnies	0	0	0
x_{12}	Cotton seed	0	0	0
x_{13}	Conc. mix Type I	0	0	0
x_{14}	Calcite	0	0	0
x_{15}	MM	0	0.0095	0.006
x_{16}	DCP	0.0131	0.0048	0.0074
x_{17}	Salt	0	0	0

Deviations	GP Model-1	GP Model-2	GP Model-3
d_{cost}^-	9.7909	10.5312	11.4146
d_{cost}^+	0	0	0
d_{CP}^-	0	0.0002	0.0001
d_{CP}^+	0	0	0
d_{TDN}^-	0	0	0
d_{TDN}^+	1.9453	1.9789	2.012
d_{Ca}^-	0.0086	0.0115	0.01
d_{Ca}^+	0	0	0
d_{Ph}^-	0.0132	0.011	0.0096
d_{Ph}^+	0.0000	0	0
d_{Rough}^-	0.0056	0.0062	0.0054
d_{Rough}^+	0.0000	0	0
d_{Conc}^-	0.0074	0.0081	0.0071
d_{Conc}^+	0.0000	0	0

Constraints	GP Model-1	GP Model-2	GP Model-3
DMI	16.75	16.89	17.03
CP	2.3524	2.395	2.4401
TDN	10.4878	10.5928	10.6973
Calcium (Ca)	0.109	0.1108	0.1107
Phosphorus (P)	0.0287	0.029	0.0304
Roughage	12.2802	12.2014	12.1431
Concentrates	4.4568	4.6743	4.8734
Least cost (z) on DM basis	116.9191	121.2922	125.2354
Objective function value	0.0127	0.0132	0.0115

5.3.4 Discussion

Table 5.11 shows the results obtained for all the goal-programming models. On assigning the weights P_1 (goal 1: cost), P_2 (goal 2: CP), P_3 (goal 3: TDN), P_4 (goal 4: Ca), P_5 (goal 5: P), P_6 (goal 6: roughage), P_7 (goal 7: concentrate) as 0.9, 0.8, 0.7, 0.6, 0.5, 0.4, 0.3 and solving the GP Model-1 using RGA with hybrid function, we obtain $d_{cost}^- = 9.7909$, $d_{TDN}^+ = 1.9453$, $d_{Ca}^- = 0.0086$, $d_{Ph}^- = 0.0132$, $d_{Rough}^- = 0.0056$, $d_{Conc}^- = 0.0074$ and the rest of the variables d_{cost}^+, d_{CP}^+, d_{CP}^-, d_{TDN}^-, d_{Ca}^+, d_{Ph}^+, d_{Rough}^+, d_{Conc}^+ as zero. We observe that goals 1, 4, 5, 6 and 7 are overachieved and goal 3 is underachieved, while goal 2 is fully achieved without any deviation, obtaining minimum $(Z) = 0.0127$. Similarly, on assigning the same weights P_1 (goal 1: cost), P_2 (goal 2: CP), P_3 (goal 3: TDN), P_4 (goal 4: Ca), P_5 (goal 5: P), P_6 (goal 6: roughage), P_7 (goal 7: concentrate) as 0.9, 0.8, 0.7, 0.6, 0.5, 0.4 and 0.3 and solving the GP Model-2 using RGA with hybrid function, we obtain $d_{cost}^- = 10.5312$, $d_{CP}^- = 0.0002$, $d_{TDN}^+ = 1.9789$, $d_{Ca}^- = 0.0115$, $d_{Ph}^- = 0.011$, $d_{Rough}^- = 0.0062$, $d_{Conc}^- = 0.0081$ and the rest of the variables d_{cost}^+, d_{CP}^+, d_{TDN}^-, d_{Ca}^+, d_{Ph}^+, d_{Rough}^+, d_{Conc}^+ as zero. Here we also observe that goals 1, 4, 5, 6 and 7 are overachieved and goal 3 is underachieved, while goal 2 is slightly overachieved, with $d_{CP}^- = 0.0002$ obtaining minimum $(Z) = 0.0132$. But on assigning the same weights P_1 (goal 1: cost), P_2 (goal 2: CP), P_3 (goal 3: TDN), P_4 (goal 4: Ca), P_5 (goal 5: P), P_6 (goal 6: roughage), P_7 (goal 7: concentrate) as 0.9, 0.8, 0.7, 0.6, 0.5, 0.4 and 0.3 and solving the GP Model-3 using RGA with hybrid function, we obtain $d_{cost}^- = 11.4146$, $d_{CP}^- = 0.0001$, $d_{TDN}^+ = 2.012$, $d_{Ca}^- = 0.01$, $d_{Ph}^- = 0.0096$, $d_{Rough}^- = 0.0054$, $d_{Conc}^- = 0.0071$ and the rest of the variables d_{cost}^+, d_{CP}^+, d_{TDN}^-, d_{Ca}^+, d_{Ph}^+, d_{Rough}^+, d_{Conc}^+ as zero. Here it is seen that goals 1, 5, 6 and 7 are overachieved and goal 3 is underachieved, while goals 2 and 4 are slightly overachieved, with deviation $d_{CP}^- = 0.0001$ and $d_{Ca}^- = 0.01$ obtaining minimum (Z) = 0.0115. The obtained result may not please the nutritionist completely; hence, he has to work on overachieved targets. The first, third, fourth, fifth, sixth and seventh goals are analysed, and the reason for the overachievement can be searched for in the diet plan. The choice of the final solution relies on the nutritionist, with, in this case, three different GP-models which represent the diet plan options that a nutritionist can choose (Babic, 2011). All possibilities are not taken into consideration, as the LP models developed in (Kuntal et al., 2016) allow introduction of additional constraints anytime, which results in a new set of solutions. Some constraints (if added) can also lead to the result of "no solution", which means that extra additional constraints are so complex that it is necessary to mediate the model by increasing some of the requirements. However, for better output, we need a further discussion with a qualified cattle nutritionist

5.3.5 Conclusion

The study focused on improving the results of the LP model developed by (Kuntal et al., 2016), formulating it into goal programming models. The GP models are solved by a real coded genetic algorithm with hybrid function to improve the quality of feed mix to the dairy cows, where this method confirms it is a useful approach in finding the low-cost diet plan for dairy cows at different body conditions. As the results obtained reveal, that RGA with hybrid function can be applied to formulate least cost rations; however, fixing the constraints and use of code for making software is considered while choosing the technique for making the least cost diet plan.

6

Study of Real Coded Hybrid Genetic Algorithm to Find Least Cost Ration for Non-Pregnant Dairy Buffaloes

CONTENTS

6.1 Introduction

In the Mandya district of Karnataka, the cost of milk per litre was more in the case of buffaloes compared to local cows due to the high fat content and high nutritive value of buffalo milk compared to its counterpart. Based on earlier research, it was clear that the productivity of the buffaloes maintained by different dairy farms was lower. Therefore, there is a need to focus on two important aspects of dairy farming: one to increase the milk productivity of buffaloes and the other one to reduce the diet cost by upgrading scientific dairy farming practices. Even though there are many predefined techniques used for animal diet formulation, a strong application of soft computing is always preferred to enhance the quality of the solution in which the rigidity in the functions as well as constraints can be easily handled by a linear programming program (LPP). Therefore, to meet the nutrient requirements at the lowest cost, we have developed a real coded hybrid genetic algorithm (RHGA) for formulating the least cost ration for dairy buffaloes, taking the hybridization of RGA and the "fmincon" of Excel Solver. This technique is better than old conventional techniques in the sense that it does not break if the inputs are modified and provides better results over complex problems even

DOI: 10.1201/9781003231714-6

if it is a linear programming model. The linear programming model is developed from primary data collected from the National Institute of Animal Nutrition and Physiology (NIANP) and as per the standards of the Indian Council of Agricultural Research (ICAR). The developed algorithms are performed equally and compared with other low-cost diet formulation techniques in non-pregnant dairy buffalo weighing 450 kg and producing 10 L of milk with 6% fat content as an LP model where standard nutrient requirements are used on a dry matter basis. Further, a goal programming model (GP model) has been developed, as there are two high priority objectives (out of eight goals) – least cost and dry matter intake – to be achieved simultaneously, if possible. This GP model is also solved by hybrid RGA, showing that four goals out of eight are fully achieved. This reveals that the real parameter-based hybrid genetic algorithm (RHGA) can be used to cut down the total mixed ration (TMR) cost without compromising the nutrient values in the diet. Although the GP model mentioned showed that 4 out of 8 goals are fully achieved, there was a concern raised about the consideration of the lower and upper bounds of the goals. Hence, a thorough review of the model in consultation with the research scientist and nutritionists from NIANP was done, and it was concluded that 7 out of 8 goals were of a maximizing nature (except least cost) within the permissible bounds, and hence the negative deviations for these seven goals should be considered in the objective function of the GP model. Only the first goal is of a minimizing nature, as it represents the cost function. Thus, a new GP model was developed for non-pregnant dairy buffalo weighing 450 kg, yielding 10 L milk with 6% of fat content that considers the standard nutrient requirement on a dry matter basis with 7 out of 8 goals as a maximization function. This model is also solved by real coded hybrid GA (RHGA), and the results obtained are in sync with reality.

In dairy farming, feeding costs account for about 70% of the total operation costs. Therefore, a different diet plan is required for different categories of buffaloes, in which the most critical part is to formulate an accurate low-cost balanced diet. While formulating the ration it is necessary to understand the nutrient requirements of buffaloes at various stages. As per the 19th Livestock Census Report of 2003, out of total livestock in the country, buffaloes are 21.2%; from 1997 to 2003, the buffalo population increased by 8.9%. As per the Ministry of Agriculture Department of Animal Husbandry, Dairying and Fisheries: Government of India, Krishi Bhavan, 19 Livestock Census–2012 All-India Report, the female buffalo population has increased by 7.99% over the previous census, and the total number of female buffaloes was 92.5 million in 2012 (www.dahd.nic.in). The buffalo population increased from 105.3 million to 108.7 million, showing a growth of 3.19%. Also, the number of milking buffaloes increased from 111.09 million to 118.59 million, an increase of 6.75% (19 Livestock Census–2012). This resulted in most of the farmers not feeding their buffaloes properly due to high feed cost and unavailability of proper feedstuffs in their respective regions, which affects the productivity of milk yield (Garg, 2012). Most of the fibrous feed available to buffaloes is deficient in essential nutrients like protein. The quantity as well as quality of feedstuffs decreases in the dry season, where farmers face a major difficulty providing a proper low-cost balanced ration to their animals in milk. Therefore, it is necessary that such lactating buffaloes should be supplemented with a balanced ration which is nutritionally rich and should be of low cost. Since 1991, many researchers have studied the feeding practices of dairy cattle, in which small farmers have limited resources for feeding and do not have proper knowledge or resources to provide a low-cost balanced ration (Leng, 1991). Study also reveals that in most of the country, animal diet is imbalanced by over-feeding energy, protein and minerals. Hence, there is a large scope for improvement in the nutritional status by adopting improved feeding practices (Mudgal et al., 2003). In addition, the dairy sector in India is highly dependent upon buffalo milk because of its contribution to total milk production (49%), as it is known that buffalo milk is rich in fat and solid content. The livestock industry plays a major role in the development of the Indian economy as the share of the livestock sector in agricultural GDP increased from 13.88% in 1980–81 to 29.20% in 2012–13 (Reddy et al., 2016) According to the Annual Report of the Department of Animal Husbandry, Dairying & Fisheries Ministry of Agriculture, Government of India (2015–16), livestock is one of the most important contributors in the Indian economy. As per the annual Report of Dept. of Animal Husbandry, Dairying and Fisheries (2016–17) India stands first in the world in milk production (155.5 million tonnes). Livestock also contribute to 4% of the national GDP (Angadi et al., 2016). A field study on the effects of feeding a balanced ration on milk production concerning nitrogen use efficiency (NUE) was conducted on 7090 lactating cows and 4534 lactating buffaloes, in which using local feed resources, a balanced least cost ration can be obtained (Garg et al., 2016). Therefore, by considering the economic importance and difficulties of Indian farmers and the importance of buffalo rearing, an improvement in feeding practices is required which results in effective milk production by optimizing the utilization of available feedstuffs and also attempts to minimize the feed cost of rations. Linear programming (LP) is a standout amongst the most normally utilized strategies followed in numerous business and non-business bolster plan programs. However, Rehman and Romero (1984) call attention to the fact that LP has numerous restrictions while detailing apportions, practically speaking. The presumptions in the LP strategy require objectives to be single and requirements to be settled on the right-hand side (RHS) (Gupta et al., 2013b). This implies the diminishment of a goal programming (GP) model comprised of limitations and a set of goals which are organized a few times. The goal of GPs is to discover the arrangement which fulfils the limitations and approach the expressed objectives of separate issues. Hypothetically, goals could be fulfilled totally, incompletely or, in some exceptional cases, not at all. This possibility is estimated utilizing positive and negative deviation factors that are characterized for every objective independently, normally known as finished or under-accomplishment of the objective. Since the target capacity of the GP plan limits the whole of the aggregate deviation from set objectives, the acquired outcome may yield a trade-off arrangement between opposing objectives (Gupta et al., 2013a). Evolutionary algorithms consist of genetic algorithm, genetic programming and their hybrid functions (Rehman [Ph.D. Thesis] 2014), and EA highly depends upon its operators (Koda, 2012). Furuya et al. in 1997 used genetic algorithms in which the ratio of ingredients evolved. In this paper, he used a new form of crossover and mutation in which mutation was generated by a combination of uniform random number and normal distribution random numbers, and the mutation rate was very high. He also solved the nonlinear constraint which showed that EA is good technique for a diet problem (Tozer and Stokes, 2001). Sahman et al. (2009) used GA to find least cost diet for a livestock, which results in good solution with few constraints.

In a nutshell we can say that appropriate feeding is the most important feature in dairy buffalo management, as the feed costs account for more than half of the total milk production (Clark and Davis, 1980). The quantity of feed that is utilized for milk production should be optimum as well as satisfy the nutrient requirement for the animal, to increase the profitability of dairy farmer. An LP model develops results with a single objective of minimizing the feed cost and rigid constraints, while converting an LP model to a GP model gives a lot of flexibility in decision making. The rigid constraints can be considered as a goal with a specific target with permissible deviations, and the solution can be seen in terms of underachievement, overachievement or fully achieved. Fixing the priorities of each goal also leads to multiple solutions, and a judicial decision can be made depending upon the preference of the dairy farmers. Since many researchers in the past addressed the issue of diet problems using EA, in this chapter, we made an effort to formulate a low-cost ration for non-pregnant buffaloes of body weight 450 kg at the third lactating period, with 10 litre milk production containing 6% fat, which was solved using an RHGA. The study was further extended to formulate nonlinear weighted goal programming models by considering the objective as the square root of the sum of the squares of the deviations.

6.2 Data Collection and Data Handling

Rations have to be formulated and need to be updated on a regular basis to avoid overfeeding. The common guidelines for diet formulation are the Indian Council of Agricultural Research (2013) and the National Research Council (2001). These provide the nutrient requirements for cow and buffaloes at different conditions (Table 6.1). An Excel-based computer program developed by NIANP in Bangalore provides actual nutrient requirement values for dry matter intake for optimizing the cost. It is difficult to optimize the cost while considering buffaloes at different conditions, so we obtained help from a qualified nutritionist while formulating the diet. A balanced diet requires frequent analyses of feedstuffs and their cost. Table 6.2 gives the selected feedstuffs for diet formulation with their nutrient values. Some variations in milk production can happen due to feeding

TABLE 6.1

Nutrient Requirements for Non-Pregnant Buffalo Weighing 450 kg and Yielding 10 Litres of Milk with 6% Fat

Total DMI (kg) min−max	CP (kg) min−max	TDN (kg) min−max	Ca (kg) min−max	Phosphorus (kg) min−max
16.42−17.24	1.7158−1.8016	7.9857−9.1835	0.0680−0.0748	0.0270−0.0405

TABLE 6.2

Nutrient Content of Feedstuffs on DM Basis

Feedstuffs	DM (in %)	CP (in kg)	TDN (in kg)	Ca (in kg)	P (in kg)	Cost C_i (in Rs)
Paddy straw	90	0.0513	0.45	0.0018	0.0008	5
CO-4 grass	20	0.08	0.52	0.0038	0.0036	3
Maize fodder	20	0.1086	0.58	0.0053	0.0014	3
Co-FS 29 sorghum	90	0.0823	0.52	0.003	0.0025	3
Ragi straw	90	0.06	0.42	0.0058	0.0025	3.5
Berseem	20	0.158	0.66	0.0144	0.0014	2
Wheat straw	90	0.033	0.55	0.003	0.0006	2
Maize stover	90	0.048	0.58	0.0053	0.0014	1.5
Maize	90	0.09	0.85	0.0053	0.0041	17
Soya DOC	90	0.46	0.7	0.0036	0.01	38
Copra DOC	90	0.27	0.7	0.002	0.009	23
Cotton DOC	90	0.35	0.7	0.0031	0.0072	23
Wheat bran	75	0.16	0.75	0.01067	0.00093	17
Gram chunnies	90	0.1645	0.7	0.0028	0.0054	14
Cotton seed	90	0.17	1.1	0.003	0.0062	21
Chickpea husk	90	0.16	0.65	0.004	0.0141	10
Conc. mix Type I	90	0.22	0.7	0.005	0.0045	17
Calcite	97	0	0	0.36	0	4
MM	90	0	0	0.32	0.06	50
DCP	90	0	0	0.24	0.16	28
Salt	90	0	0	0	0	5

practices, availability of feed resources or animal grouping factors. Roughages and concentrates which are rich in digestibility should be used in the correct proportion depending upon the lactation period and the quantity of milk with a high percentage of fat, so depending upon conditions the roughage–concentrate ration can vary. To obtain the least cost feed we have some constraints for each nutrient, and it is unique for each animal. The minimum and maximum levels of crude protein (CP 10.4–11%), total digestible nutrient (TDN 48.6–51.1%), calcium (0.4–0.5%) and phosphorus (0.16–0.18%) can be met through different proportions of roughage (40–80%) and concentrates (20–70%) on total dry matter intake for milking buffalo.

6.3 Problem Description

The present study computes the balanced least cost ration for buffalo of body weight 450 kg in the third lactation period, where buffalo need a ration for body maintenance with 10 litres of milk production (6% fat content). The nutrient requirements of buffalo are calculated by an Excel-based computer program developed

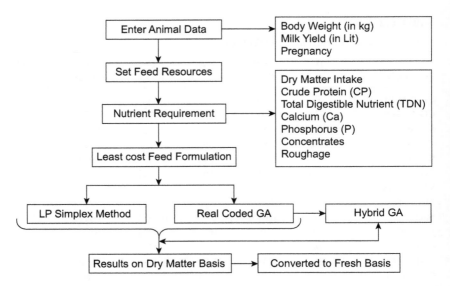

FIGURE 6.1 Methodology to Calculate Least Cost Balanced Ration for Non-Pregnant Dairy Buffalo; Kuntal, Adv in Intelligent System & Computing, 2017.

by NIANP, Bangalore, as per the ICAR 2013 and NRC 2001 standard. A linear programming model is introduced for the specified condition of buffalo. Although there is a well-defined method to solve LPP, an evolutionary algorithm (EA) is preferable, as these algorithms efficiently deal with the mathematical rigidity of the constraints, can handle large dimension problems and also give multiple solutions. Since the number of variables represented as feedstuffs are greater in number and the constraints are very rigid, we opted to develop an RHGA to solve the ration formulation problem for buffaloes. Various versions of this algorithm were created, and a comparative study was planned to obtain the appropriate method which can be used by the farmers at farm level.

6.3.1 Linear Programming Model

Objective Function: Min(z) $= \sum_{i=1}^{21} C_i x_i$

Subjected to:

1. $16.42\,\text{Kg} \leq \sum_{i=1}^{21} x_i \leq 17.42\,\text{Kg}$
2. $1.7158\,\text{Kg} \leq \sum_{i=1}^{21} CP_i \leq 1.8016\,\text{Kg}$

3. $7.9857 \text{Kg} \leq \sum_{i=1}^{21} \text{TDN}_i \leq 9.1835 \text{Kg}$

4. $0.0680 \text{Kg} \leq \sum_{i=1}^{21} \text{Ca}_i \leq 0.0748 \text{Kg}$

5. $0.0270 \text{Kg} \leq \sum_{i=1}^{21} \text{Ph}_i \leq 0.0405 \text{Kg}$

6. $6.568 \text{Kg} \leq \sum_{i=1}^{8} \text{Rough}_i \leq 13.136 \text{Kg}$

7. $3.224 \text{Kg} \leq \sum_{i=9}^{21} \text{Conc}_i \leq 11.494 \text{Kg}$

Search Space:

$0.806 \leq x_1 \leq 4.03, 0.806 \leq x_2 \leq 4.03, 0.806 \leq x_3 \leq 4.03, 0.806 \leq x_4 \leq 4.03, 0.806$
$\leq x_5 \leq 4.03, 0.806 \leq x_6 \leq 3.224, 0.806 \leq x_7 \leq 3.224, 0.806 \leq x_8 \leq 4.03,$
$0.806 \leq x_9 \leq 3.224, 0 \leq x_{10} \leq 4.03, 0 \leq x_{11} \leq 4.03, 0 \leq x_{12} \leq 3.2240,$
$0 \leq x_{13} \leq 3.224, 0.1612 \leq x_{14} \leq 0.806, 0.1612 \leq x_{15} \leq 0.806, 0.0806 \leq x_{16} \leq 0.806,$
$0.806 \leq x_{17} \leq 3.224, 0 \leq x_{18} \leq 0.1612, 0, 0 \leq x_{19} \leq 0.0806, 0 \leq x_{20} \leq 0.03224,$
$0.12896 \leq x_{21} \leq 0.1612$

6.3.2 Goal Programming Model-1

$$Min(Z) = \sqrt{\begin{array}{l} p_1 \left(d_{cost}^+\right)^2 + p_2 \left(d_{DM}^+\right)^2 + p_3 \left(d_{CP}^+\right)^2 + p_4 \left(d_{TDN}^+\right)^2 + p_5 \left(d_{Ca}^+\right)^2 \\ + p_6 \left(d_{Ph}^+\right)^2 + p_7 \left(d_{Rough}^+\right)^2 + p_8 \left(d_{Conc}^+\right)^2 \end{array}}$$

Subjected to:

1. Goal 1 (minimize Least Cost): $\sum_{i=1}^{21} C_i x_i + d_{cost}^- - d_{cost}^+ = 101.6073$

2. Goal 2 (minimize Dry Matter): $\sum_{i=1}^{21} x_i + d_{DM}^- - d_{DM}^+ = 16.42 \text{ Kg}$

3. Goal 3 (minimize Crude Protein): $\sum_{i=1}^{21} CP_i + d_{CP}^- - d_{CP}^+ = 1.7158 \text{ Kg}$

4. Goal 4 (minimize Total Digestible Nutrient): $\sum_{i=1}^{21} TDN_i + d_{TDN}^- - d_{TDN}^+$
   $= 9.1835 \text{ Kg}$

5. Goal 5 (minimize Calcium): $\sum_{i=1}^{21} Ca_i + d_{Ca}^- - d_{Ca}^+ = 0.0748 \text{ Kg}$

6. Goal 6 (minimize Phosphorus): $\sum_{i=1}^{21} Ph_i + d_{Ph}^- - d_{Ph}^+ = 0.0405 \text{ Kg}$

7. Goal 7 (minimize Roughages): $\sum_{i=1}^{21} Rough_i + d_{Rough}^- - d_{Rough}^+$
   $= 13.136 \text{ Kg}$

8. Goal 8 (minimize Concentrates): $\sum_{i=1}^{21} Conc_i + d_{Conc}^- - d_{Conc}^+ = 3.2840 \text{ Kg}$

TABLE 6.3

Priority Values for GP Model-1

Priorities	Goals	Value
p_1	Min least cost	0.9
p_2	Min DM	0.8
p_3	Min CP	0.7
p_4	Min TDN	0.6
p_5	Min Ca	0.5
p_6	Min P	0.4
p_7	Min roughage	0.3
p_8	Min concentrate	0.2

TABLE 6.4

Priority Values for GP Model-2

Priorities	Goals	Value
p_1	Min least cost	0.9
p_2	Min DM	0.8

6.3.3 Goal Programming Model-2

$$Min(Z) = \sqrt{p_1\left(d_{cost}^{+}\right)^2 + p_2\left(d_{DM}^{+}\right)^2}$$

Subjected to:

1. Goal 1 (minimize Least Cost): $\sum_{i=1}^{21} C_i x_i + d_{cost}^{-} - d_{cost}^{+} = 101.6073$
2. Goal 2 (minimize Dry Matter): $\sum_{i=1}^{21} x_i + d_{DM}^{-} - d_{DM}^{+} = 16.42$ Kg

6.3.4 Goal Programming Model-3 (Auxiliary Approach)

$$Min(Z) = \sqrt{\begin{array}{l} p_1\left(d_{cost}^{+}\right)^2 + p_2\left(d_{CP}^{-}\right)^2 + p_3\left(d_{TDN}^{-}\right)^2 + p_4\left(d_{Ca}^{-}\right)^2 + p_5\left(d_{Ph}^{-}\right)^2 \\ + p_6\left(d_{Rough}^{-}\right)^2 + p_7\left(d_{Conc}^{-}\right)^2 \end{array}}$$

Subjected to:

1. Goal 1 (Minimize Least Cost): $\sum_{i=1}^{21} C_i x_i + d_{cost}^{-} - d_{cost}^{+} = 101.6073$
2. Goal 2 (Maximize Crude Protein): $\sum_{i=1}^{21} CP_i + d_{CP}^{-} - d_{CP}^{+} = 1.7158$ Kg

3. Goal 3 (Maximize Total Digestible Nutrient): $\sum_{i=1}^{21} TDN_i + d_{TDN}{}^{-}$

   $-d_{TDN}{}^{+} = 9.1835$ Kg

4. Goal 4 (Maximize Calcium): $\sum_{i=1}^{21} Ca_i + d_{Ca}{}^{-} - d_{Ca}{}^{+} = 0.0748$ Kg

5. Goal 5 (Maximize Phosphorus): $\sum_{i=1}^{21} Ph_i + d_{Ph}{}^{-} - d_{Ph}{}^{+} = 0.0405$ Kg

6. Goal 6 (Maximize Roughages): $\sum_{i=1}^{8} Rough_i + d_{Rough}{}^{-} - d_{Rough}{}^{+}$

   $= 13.136$ Kg

7. Goal 7 (Maximize Concentrates): $\sum_{i=1}^{21} Conc_i + d_{Conc}{}^{-} - d_{Conc}{}^{+}$

   $= 3.2840$ Kg

8. $\sum_{i=1}^{21} x_i = 16.42$ Kg

where p_i ($I = 1,2\ldots.7$) are positive numbers between $(0,1)$ such that $p_1 > p_2 > \ldots p_7$

6.4 Development of Real Coded Hybrid Genetic Algorithm

A genetic algorithm (GA) is a heuristic based technique which is based on evolutionary theory. GA works on a solution space instead of a state space, where it builds new solutions based on existing ones. GA combines good portions of the solution just as nature does by combining the DNA of living beings. To use a GA, first we create an initial population, then we decide the "gene" representation; we chose default population type "double vector" to represent genes due to its flexibility. After selecting the representation of genes, the population undergoes three main operators of GA such as selection, crossover and mutation operators to create the next generation from current generations. In brief, a selection operator selects parents that combine to populate the next generation. The crossover operator also combines two parents to create new offspring for the next generation, and the mutation operator randomly changes the individuals to create new offspring. MATLAB provides "gaoptimset" to create or modify the GA option structure.

6.4.1 Objective Function, Decision Variables, Representation of Plots

Firstly, we provide the objective function, that is, the function that calculates minimum cost of ration of each member of population. In our linear model, we have 21 decision variables and 14 constraints from which we have to find the minimum cost; hence, we set the number of variables to 21. We used "gaoptimset" for representation of population. Population type specifies the type of input to the fitness function, so we have restricted the input to population as "double vector" since we do not have complex decision variables. We used some plot options in "gaoptimset" such as @gaplotbestf, @gaplotdistance and @gaplotrange to see the performance of population in each generation, where "gaplotbestf" plots the best fitness value in each generation and "gaplotdistance" plots the average distance between individuals by taking 20 samples at every generation. It calculates the distance of each sample and stores the choice, then calculates the average distance by using mean square error. The performance of GA will be affected by the diversity of the initial population if the distance between populations is large, the diversity is large; if the distance is low, the diversity is less. More trials are required to experiment with the right amount of diversity because if the diversity is too high or low, GA will not perform well and the solution may stick to local minimum. We have created the population in the range of lower and upper bounds and tried to program the GA to search in that space. Population size determines the size of population at each generation; hence, we have selected four times the number of variables to perform in every generation. Obviously, by increasing the population size, the GA will perform better by searching more points and is more likely to provide a better solution. In this case, we have rigid constraints and bounds; therefore, by increasing the population size, it will take a long time for the GA to generate the population.

6.4.2 Crossover, Selection, Mutation and Elitism Operators

The selection operator in a GA selects best fit parents to perform crossover and mutation. In a tournament selection, every individual is chosen randomly to perform in the tournament based on tournament size, and then the best fit individual is selected as a parent. We chose tournament size as two. In a crossover operator, two parents are combined to form offspring for the next iterations. A heuristic crossover is chosen, as offspring moves from worst parents to the previous best parent, for example, if P_1 and P_2 are parents and P_1 has better fitness then offspring $= P_2 + 1.2 \times (P_1 - P_2)$, where 1.2 is the ratio to perform the heuristic crossover. Mutation decides how the algorithm makes small changes in the individuals randomly to create the mutation offspring. It is an important parameter of the algorithm because it provides diversity that allows the GA to search in a broader space. We have rigid linear constraints and bounds; hence, from the GA options an adaptive feasible mutation was preferred. These mutation options are better for linear constraints and bounds as they creates direction which is very flexible with regard to previous favorable or unfavorable generations (repository.um.edu). A best fit region called a feasible region is restricted by the linear equality and inequality constraints; therefore, to satisfy these constraints, a step length is chosen towards the direction.

6.4.3 Global vs. Local Minima

After specifying these genetic algorithm options for linear models, many times a GA gives local minima instead of global minima (rad.inu.edu.gr). Therefore, to overcome this deficiency of the GA we have introduced the hybrid command "fmincon" inside the GA, in which we allow GA to find the valley that contains the global minimum, and after the last generation, it takes the last value of GA as the initial value of "fmincon" to converge quickly. Also, one can try to test GA in the wider range by increasing the diversity of the initial population by manipulating the initial population. However, we have rigid constraints and bounds, so we want to search the point in the specified lower and upper bounds only. "Fmincon" is a gradient-based search technique which works on a problem with continuous constraints and objective functions and must have a first derivative. In MATLAB, "fmincon" uses a sequential quadratic programming (SQP) sub-problem where SQP methods are a representation of nonlinear programming methods. Schittkowski (Singh and Singh, 2015) has executed a version that surpasses every other tested method in terms of efficiency and accuracy of the solution for a large number of test problems (tel.archives-ouvertes.fr). Based on previous work (Biggs, 1975; Han, 1977; Powell, 1978a), it can be seen that the method mimics Newton's method for a constrained problem. At every generation, an initial judgment is made of the Hessian of the Lagrangian function using a quasi-Newton method, which is used to generate a quadratic programming (QP) problem whose solution is a benchmark which is used to form a search direction for a line search problem (tel.archives-ouvertes.fr). A major overview of SQP is discussed in (Fletcher, 1987; Gill et al., 1981; Powell, 1978b; Hock and Schittkowski, 1983). In light of this, we have used the SQP algorithm for "fmincon" Solver, where the SQP algorithm (identical to SQP–legacy algorithm) is the same as the active-set algorithm but has a different implementation. An interior point algorithm can also be used, but SQP has faster execution time and less memory usage then the SQP-legacy and interior point algorithms. Nocedal and Wright explain the basic SQP algorithm (Nocedal and Wright, 2006).

6.5 Results on Dry Matter and As-Fresh Basis

TABLE 6.5

Least Cost Ration Formulated by Various Techniques for Non-Pregnant Dairy Buffalo on DM Basis (LP Model)

	Minimum value obtained in 10 runs for 5000 generations			RGA with hybrid function
Feedstuffs	**RGA without crossover**	**RGA without mutation**	**RGA with crossover and mutation**	
Paddy straw	3.7907	3.8114	3.187	2.363
CO-4 grass	0.8758	0.806	1.3551	0.806
Maize fodder	2.3054	2.7951	2.0736	3.086
Co-Fs 29 sorghum	1.3639	0.806	1.112	2.266
Ragi straw	1.7162	1.5121	2.0725	2.197
Berseem	1.2667	0.806	0.9759	0.806
Wheat straw	0.9611	1.601	0.8703	0.806
Maize stover	0.8572	0.806	1.3561	0.806
Maize	0.8060	0.806	0.8061	0.806
Soya DOC	0.0001	0.5647	0.0057	0

(Continued)

TABLE 6.5

(Continued)

	Minimum value obtained in 10 runs for 5000 generations			RGA with hybrid function
Feedstuffs	RGA without crossover	RGA without mutation	RGA with crossover and mutation	
Copra DOC	0.0015	0	0.0101	0
Cotton DOC	1.1233	0.4301	1.2101	0.951
Wheat bran	0.0003	0	0.0114	0
Cotton seed	0.1613	0.1612	0.1612	0.161
Chickpea husk	0.0855	0.0806	0.0911	0.081
Conc. mix Type-I	0.8076	0.806	0.8258	0.963
Calcite	0.0017	0.0117	0.0007	0
MM	0	0	0	0
DCP	0	0	0	0
Salt	0.1322	0.1612	0.129	0.161
DMI	16.419	16.42	16.419	16.42
CP	1.7148	1.7148	1.7151	1.7158
TDN	9.175	9.1835	9.1816	9.1835
Calcium (Ca)	0.0758	0.0746	0.075	0.0748
Phosphorus (P)	0.0388	0.0391	0.0412	0.0405
Roughage	13.137	12.9436	13.0025	13.1360
Concentrates	3.282	3.4765	3.4165	3.2840
Least cost (z)	104.8323	113.7639	106.0145	101.6073

6.6 Discussion

The results obtained by various techniques – viz. RGA without crossover, RGA without mutation, RGA with crossover and mutation and RGA with hybrid function – for least cost ration for dairy buffalo (which is run 10 times up to 5000 generations) are presented in Table 6.5. The LP model for dairy buffalo has 21 variables, which are too complex for finding an optimal solution. RGA is also a heuristic technique, which works on a principle of survival of best fit and tournament selection. Adaptive feasibility mutation and heuristic crossover are used along with elitism to solve the LP model for dairy buffalo. Although RGA without crossover, RGA without mutation and RGA with crossover and mutation give a near-optimal answer, we provide a solution using RGA with hybrid function to avoid the solution being stuck in local minima. As farmers need a total mixed ration to feed dairy buffalo on as fresh basis, we have converted the least cost and total mixed ration obtained by all techniques to as fresh basis, and the results are given in Table 6.6. As per Table 6.5, this category of animals requires about 16.42 kg of dry matter from various kinds of feeds, which should contain 1715.8 g of protein, 9183.5 g of TDN, 74.8g of calcium and 40.5 g of phosphorus. These nutrient requirements can be met from 13.13 kg of roughage and 3.28 kg of concentrates on dry matter, amounting to Rupees 101.6703 per day per cattle on dry matter basis. As fresh basis is a feed nutrient content with moisture included. After converting to as fresh basis, feedstuffs required for dairy buffalo are approximately 36.3 kg per day, amounting to Rs 4.52 per kg using the RGA with hybrid function. When the expected nutrient requirement solution was sought using RGA without crossover, without mutation and with crossover and mutation, the least cost ration obtained was Rs 4.59 per kg, Rs 4.93 per kg and Rs 4.67 per kg, respectively. The detailed analysis of the ration is showed in Tables 6.5 and 6.6 which exactly meets the requirements of dry matter, CP, TDN, calcium and phosphorus. The requirements of roughage and concentrates are also met within the permissible range. In addition, results obtained by GP Model-1, 2 and 3 are shown in Tables 6.7, 6.8 and 6.9, which reveals that from GP-1 goals 5 and 8 are fully achieved and goals 1, 2, 3, 4, 6 and 7 are underachieved. The least cost obtained by GP-1 is Rs 100.79 on DM basis, but DMI and CP were not satisfied. Whereas by GP Model-2, our high priorities,

TABLE 6.6

Least Cost Ration Formulated by Various Techniques for Non-Pregnant Dairy Buffalo on "As Fresh Basis" (LP Model)

Feedstuffs	RGA without crossover	RGA without mutation	RGA with crossover and mutation	RGA with hybrid function
Paddy straw	4.211889	4.234889	3.541111	2.625556
CO-4 grass	4.379	4.03	6.7755	4.03
Maize fodder	11.527	13.9755	10.368	15.43
Co-FS 29 sorghum	1.515444	0.895556	1.235556	2.517778
Ragi straw	1.906889	1.680111	2.302778	2.441111
Berseem	6.3335	4.03	4.8795	4.03
Wheat straw	1.067889	1.778889	0.967	0.895556
Maize stover	0.952444	0.895556	1.506778	0.895556
Maize	0.895556	0.895556	0.895667	0.895556
Soya DOC	0.000111	0.627444	0.006333	0
Copra DOC	0.001667	0	0.011222	0
Cotton DOC	1.248111	0.477889	1.344556	1.056667
Wheat bran	0.0004	0	0.0152	0
Gram chunnies	0.180444	0.505444	0.183556	0.178889
Cotton seed	0.179222	0.179111	0.179111	0.178889
Chickpea husk	0.095	0.089556	0.101222	0.09
Conc. mix Type I	0.897333	0.895556	0.917556	1.07
Calcite	0.001753	0.012062	0.000722	0
MM	0	0	0	0
DCP	0	0	0	0
Salt	0.146889	0.179111	0.143333	0.178889
TMR on as fresh basis in kg	35.5405415	35.3822285	35.3746994	36.33556
Least cost in Rs on as fresh basis	163.445699	174.679247	165.425231	164.5728
Least cost (Rs per kg)	4.59885225	4.93692045	4.67637135	4.529249

TABLE 6.7

Least Cost and Deviation Value Solved by Hybrid RGA for GP Model-1

Feedstuffs	Values
On dry matter basis	
Paddy straw	3.5806
CO-4 grass	0.1175
Maize fodder	0.0194
Co-FS 29 sorghum	0.1334
Ragi straw	1.0355
Berseem	2.7540
Wheat straw	2.6429
Maize stover	0.5415
Maize	1.3333
Soya DOC	1.0162
Copra DOC	0.0146
Cotton DOC	0.0240
Wheat bran	0
Gram chunnies	0.0107
Cotton seed	0
Chickpea husk	0.0214
Conc. mix Type I	0
Calcite	0
MM	0
DCP	0
Salt	0.8638
Deviations	
d_{cost}^-	0.8115
d_{cost}^+	0
d_{DM}^-	2.3113
d_{DM}^+	0
d_{CP}^-	0.2942
d_{CP}^+	0
d_{TDN}^-	1.5173
d_{TDN}^+	0
d_{Ca}^-	0
d_{Ca}^+	0
d_{Ph}^-	0.0118
d_{Ph}^+	0
d_{Rough}^-	2.3113
d_{Rough}^+	0
d_{Conc}^-	0
d_{Conc}^+	0
DMI	14.1088
CP	1.4216

Feedstuffs	Values
TDN	7.6663
Calcium (Ca)	0.0748
Phosphorus (P)	0.0287
Roughage	10.8248
Concentrates	3.2840
Least cost on DM basis	100.7965
As fresh basis	
TMR on as fresh basis in kg	26.91883
Least cost in Rs on as fresh basis	135.0133
Least cost (in Rs per kg)	5.015569

TABLE 6.8

Least Cost and Deviation Value Solved by Hybrid RGA for GP Model-2

Feedstuffs	Values
On dry matter basis	
Paddy straw	1.1775
CO-4 grass	0.9571
Maize fodder	0.0001
Co-FS 29 sorghum	5.7964
Ragi straw	0
Berseem	2.5561
Wheat straw	2.6487
Maize stover	0
Maize	0
Soya DOC	0.8576
Copra DOC	0
Cotton DOC	0.0001
Wheat bran	0
Gram chunnies	0
Cotton seed	1.2705
Chickpea husk	0
Conc. mix Type I	0
Calcite	0
MM	0
DCP	0
Salt	1.1559
Deviations	
d_{cost}^-	0.0001
d_{cost}^+	0
d_{DM}^-	0
d_{DM}^+	0

(*Continued*)

TABLE 6.8

(Continued)

Feedstuffs	Values
d_{CP}^-	0.0032
d_{CP}^+	0.0997
d_{TDN}^-	0.2440
d_{TDN}^+	1.5679
d_{Ca}^-	0.0055
d_{Ca}^+	0.2868
d_{Ph}^-	0.0663
d_{Ph}^+	0.7203
d_{Rough}^-	0.0216
d_{Rough}^+	0.0182
d_{Conc}^-	0.2544
d_{Conc}^+	0.0095
DMI	16.4200
CP	1.7158
TDN	9.1835
Calcium (Ca)	0.0748
Phosphorus (P)	0.0405
Roughage	13.1359
Concentrates	3.2841
Least cost on DM basis	101.6090
As fresh basis	
TMR on as fresh basis in kg	30.62294
Least cost in Rs on as fresh basis	143.947
Least cost (in Rs per kg)	4.700626

TABLE 6.9

Least Cost and Deviation Value Solved by Hybrid RGA for GP Model-3

Feedstuffs	Values
On dry matter basis	
Paddy straw	0.0272
CO-4 grass	0
Maize fodder	0
Co-FS 29 sorghum	0
Ragi straw	0.0171
Berseem	13.074
Wheat straw	0.0156
Maize stover	0.0022
Maize	0.0505
Soya DOC	0
Copra DOC	0.0053

Feedstuffs	Values
Cotton DOC	0.0006
Wheat bran	0.0227
Gram chunnies	0.0231
Cotton seed	0.4741
Chickpea husk	0.0151
Conc. mix Type I	0.0057
Calcite	1.4125
MM	1.1399
DCP	0.0001
Salt	0.1344
Deviations	
d_{cost}^-	0.0021
d_{cost}^+	0
d_{CP}^-	0
d_{CP}^+	0.4508
d_{TDN}^-	0
d_{TDN}^+	0.0901
d_{Ca}^-	0
d_{Ca}^+	0.9891
d_{Ph}^-	0
d_{Ph}^+	0.0499
d_{Rough}^-	0
d_{Rough}^+	0
d_{Conc}^-	0
d_{Conc}^+	0
DMI	16.4200
CP	2.1666
TDN	9.2736
Calcium (Ca)	1.0639
Phosphorus (P)	0.0904
Roughage	13.1360
Concentrates	3.2840
Least cost on DM basis	101.6052
As fresh basis	
TMR on as fresh basis in kg	68.97967
Least cost in Rs on as fresh basis	214.2146
Least cost (in Rs per kg)	3.105474

goals 1 and 2, are completely satisfied and the rest of the goals are either under-achieved or overachieved, but the least cost obtained was Rs 100.6090 per day per cattle on dry matter basis, which is same as the LP model. The amount of feedstuffs is much less compared to the LP model, which is truly an advantage to farmers because of the limitation of feedstuff. From a farmer's point of view, the TMR required for the farmer by the RGA hybrid function is 26.9 kg per day, amounting to Rs 5.01 per kg, whereas by GP Model-2, the TMR required is 30 kg per day, amounting to approximately Rs 4.7 per kg, which is less compared to the RGA hybrid function. However, for a better output for farmers, we need a further discussion with a qualified cattle nutritionist. For GP Model-3, we observe that on assigning the weights P_1 (goal 1: cost), P_2 (goal 2: CP), P_3 (goal 3: TDN), P_4 (goal 4: Ca), P_5 (goal 5: P), P_6 (goal 6: roughage), P_7 (goal 7: concentrate) as 0.9, 0.8, 0.7, 0.6, 0.5, 0.4 and 0.3 and solving the GP Model using RGA with hybrid function, we obtain $d_{cost}^- = 0.0021$, $d_{CP}^+ = 0.4508$, $d_{TDN}^+ = 0.0901$, $d_{Ca}^+ = 0.9891$, $d_{Ph}^+ = 0.0499$, and rest of the deviational variables d_{cost}^+, d_{CP}^-, d_{TDN}^-, d_{Ca}^-, d_{Ph}^-, d_{Rough}^-, d_{Rough}^+, d_{Conc}^-, d_{Conc}^+ are zero. We observe that goal 1 is overachieved, goals 2, 3, 4 and 5 are underachieved and goals 6 and 7 are fully achieved without any deviation with minimum $(Z) = 0$. The results obtained in this work are better than the results obtained for GP Model-1. On comparing the results obtained in both the models, d_{cost}^-, d_{DM}^-, d_{CP}^-, d_{TDN}^-, d_{Ph}^-, d_{Rough}^- are overachieved, while d_{Ca}^-, d_{Ca}^+, d_{Conc}^-, d_{Conc}^+ are fully achieved, due to which all constraints except calcium and concentrates are satisfied with the least cost of Rs 100.605/- on DM basis. The reason for not satisfying the constraints by the goal programming model is adding the deviation variables to dry matter basis; that is, dry matter intake is one of the fixed constraints, and hence it has to be treated as a constraint rather than treating it simply as a goal. In the present work, after considering all the loopholes, a new goal-programming model has been developed which gives an improved solution in which almost all the constraints are satisfied including our high priority goals (least cost and dry matter intake). The obtained result was not completely accepted by the nutritionist, as the reasons for underachieved and overachieved targets need to be analysed, because the choice of a final solution depends on the nutritionist, and there is a need of further discussion with the nutritionist for better output.

6.7 Conclusion

The present study addresses the use of a real coded genetic algorithm with hybrid function (RHGA) as a tool to provide a good quality feed mix to the dairy buffalo for better health and milk production. All the techniques – viz. RGA without crossover, RGA without Mutation, RGA with crossover and mutation and RGA with hybrid function – for the least cost ration are performing equally. RGA without crossover and RGA without mutation operator provide near-optimal answers, but the solutions seem to be get stuck in local minima; hence, it is proved that the real coded genetic algorithm with hybrid function (RHGA) provides an optimal solution, and this method can be used effectively for a low-cost diet plan for dairy buffalo. Nutrient requirements of buffalo are calculated by an Excel-based computer program developed by NIANP, Bangalore, as per the Indian Council of Agricultural Research–ICAR 2013 and NRC 2001 standard. Application of the RHGA in solving GP Model-1, 2 and 3 for the ration formulation problem of Indian buffaloes in the Mandya district of Karnataka is found to be very efficient. Further detailed research with various species of animals and with different physiological needs may be required to fine-tune the techniques for farmers' use. In addition to that, we are able to cut down the cost of TMR without any nutrient deficiency in the diet.

7

Conclusion

The main purpose of formulating the diet problem is to find the combination of feed ingredients which satisfies the entire daily nutritional requirements of dairy animals with minimum cost. As the farmer's objective is to reduce the cost of ration and to maximize the profit, since spending more on rations will decrease the profitability of farmer, this can be achieved by scientific and economic efficiency. This study is the proof that optimization of the ration at a cheaper rate is possible at different body conditions of dairy cows and buffaloes by combining linear and goal programming (LP and GP) with priority functions and using a heuristic technique called a real coded genetic algorithm (RGA). The entire idea was first tested with a nonlinear model for Sahiwal cows with the objective of maximizing the milk yield by Pratiksha Sexena using a binary coded genetic algorithm. The effectiveness of the binary coded genetic algorithm was also tested on three linear programming model and a nonlinear goal programming model extracted from the work of Shrabani Gosh, where these mathematical models are developed for different conditions, viz: if a fully grown cow having a body weight of 500 kg:

    i. Does not produce milk,
   ii. Produces different levels of milk with a certain amount of fat,
  iii. Is pregnant in the third trimester, where it needs extra nutrient supplements.

Later, three linear programming (LP) models and nonlinear programming (NLP) models are formulated for the least cost diet of dairy cows of body weight 500 kg, where the cows during pregnancy at third trimester need a balanced ration for body maintenance, milk production (with a minimum of 4% of fat content) and for fetus growth. These models are solved by an RGA (with and without seeding the random number generation), and the results are compared with Excel Solver tools, namely GRG nonlinear, evolutionary algorithm (EA) and simplex LP. Further, the study has been extended to the development of linear and goal programming models of non-pregnant dairy buffalo of body weight 450 kg, which need a ration to produce 10 litres of milk with 6% fat content. It has been observed that in all these case studies, reductions of ration cost is possible by heuristic techniques as compared to the old conventional method, irrespective of the rigidity of constraints. For better diet formulation, the minimum and maximum range (in percentage) of crude protein (CP), total digestible nutrients (TDN), dry matter (DM), calcium, phosphorus, roughage and concentrates are introduced in both LP and GP models based on ICAR 2013 and NRC 2001 standards. The RGA and hybrid genetic algorithm (RHGA)

DOI: 10.1201/9781003231714-7

were developed to overcome the limitation of binary coded GA. In Chapter 4, we considered the case study in which Pratiksha Sexena solved a nonlinear model using the Kuhn-Tucker method, which resulted in the values of three nutrient ingredients, CP, TDM and DM as $x_1 = 782.97800$, $x_2 = 67.00717$ and $x_3 = 507.79209$ gm/kg metabolic body weight, with the maximum objective value of 582.01gm/kg metabolic weight. Results obtained for the three nutrients using the genetic algorithm for the nonlinear model with the original bounds is $x_1 = (721.3220, 747.1494)$, $x_2 = (71.5456, 74.6055)$, $x_3 = (432.3138, 474.6072)$ gm/kg metabolic body weight, with maximum objective value of 819.1805 gm/kg metabolic weight (Gupta et al., 2013b). For reduced bounds, the wide range of solutions obtained is $x_1 = (670.5081, 677.1270)$, $x_2 = (68.8769, 69.4029)$, $x_3 = (428.7671, 463.4859)$ gm/kg metabolic weight, with the global maxima of 593.8254 gm/kg metabolic weight (Gupta et al., 2013b). Further, the nonlinear model was also solved by controlled random search technique (RST2) with original and reduced bounds, which revealed that variations in the value of decision variables x_1, x_2 and x_3 are 4.3%, −0.19% and 20.17%, respectively, which leads to 0.68% variation in maximum milk yield (objective function). There is approximately 2% deviation in the objective function compared to the Kuhn-Tucker method. Therefore, the solution of NLPP (1) and (2) using a genetic algorithm reveals that the variation of decision variables x_1, x_2 and x_3 are 9.3%, 6.9% and 6.08%, respectively, which leads to a 27% variation in the objective function and is more compared to RST2 (Gupta et al., 2013b). Using a wide range of bounds for GA, results were obtained only after 3000 generations, whereas after reducing the bounds the best result is obtained in 500 generations. Hence, reduction of bounds gives the better result. After comparing the results obtained by GA with RST2, it reveals that both techniques are comparable, with a small deviation of 4.6%. Therefore, there is a possibility of solving the nonlinear model of animal diet using GA with a slight modification in the technique according to the requirement of the planner. GA gives flexibility to choose any option from the wide range of solutions that act as an additional bonus to the planner.

The second case study in Chapter 4 is extracted from the work of Shrabani Gosh, which consists of three nonlinear goal programming models for Level-1, 2 and 3 to test the effect of a binary genetic algorithm on animal diet formulation. The focus was to discuss the results of deviational variables obtained by binary coded genetic algorithm developed by Mitsuo Gen et al. (1997) rather than discussing the details of model formulation. This study reveals that the GA approach gives better results as compared to RST (see Figure 4.7). It is also noticed from the results shown in Table 4.7 that goal 1 and goal 15 were overachieved for Level-1. In Level-2, goal 16 is overachieved, and in Level-3, goal 1 is overachieved. All other goals are fully achieved in a thousand generations using GA for the linear model. Figure 4.5 can be referred to see the wholistic view of the goals' achievements. Figure 4.6 displays the goals' achievement levels for a nonlinear model. We can see that goal 1 and goal 15 are overachieved for Level-1. In Level-2, all the goals are achieved, and for Level-3, goal 1 and goal 16 are overachieved. All other goals are fully achieved in 1000 generations using GA for a nonlinear model. Therefore, it can be concluded that by fine-tuning the nutritive goals and by introducing harmless deviations as underachievement and overachievement, binary coded genetic algorithm can be applied effectively for finding the least cost diet plan. In addition, after analysing the approach applied by Shrabani Ghosh, it was found that minerals are not used while formulating the diet plan. But there are three different body conditions of animals, which definitely requires additional nutrient supplements called minerals, and this supplement cannot be obtained from feedstuffs.

In Chapter 5, we took into account this important aspect of including minerals as essential nutrient requirement for the animal while formulating the diet plan for cattle in the Mandya district of Karnataka. Using the primary data of the Mandya district of Karnataka, taken from NIANP Bangalore, three different linear models were formulated for dairy cattle with body weight 500 kg and a 10 litre milk yield with 4% of fat content who were in the seventh, eighth and ninth months of pregnancy. The constraints for these LP models are fixed by giving a minimum and maximum percentage range on dry matter basis, which was not considered by researchers earlier. This feature makes the model easy to understand, but at the same time the model becomes rigid. The minimum and maximum level of CP is 9.82–11%, TDN is 46.73–51%, calcium is 0.38–0.8%, phosphorus is 0.23–0.5%, roughage is 40–80% and concentrate is 20–70%, as calculated on total DMI for each type of cattle. These LP models are solved using LP simplex, GRG nonlinear, evolutionary algorithm (EA) and real coded genetic algorithm (RGA) with seeding the random numbers. The LP simplex method provides an iterative algorithm to locate the corner points systematically until we get an optimal solution. The GRG nonlinear algorithm with forward differencing deals with problems involving decision variables and nonlinear constraints. Forward differencing uses a single point that is slightly different from the current value to find the derivative. Solving LP models in Excel Solver, it will not compute derivatives again and again, and it continues to estimate the solution along the straight line instead of recalculating the changing gradients. When GRG finds a solution, this means that Solver has found a valley for minimizing the objective function after satisfying the Karush-Kuhn-Tucker (KKT) conditions for local optimality, and there are no other possible solutions for decision variables (feedstuffs) near to current values. EA is also used to solve the LP model by seeding the random number generator. The results obtained by various techniques for LP models, are presented in Tables 5.4, 5.6 and 5.8 for Cattle-1, 2 and 3 on DM basis. LP models 1, 2 and 3 have 17 decision variables and eight constraints with minimum and maximum range. In this study, the EA method with seeding technique could not find least cost because costlier nutrients like the crude protein level in final feed was higher (1.82 kg) in EA as compared to other method (1.644 kg). Similarly, TDN content is also higher in the EA method than other methods. These could be the reasons for higher costs (INR 163.14) obtained using EA compared to other methods (GRG–126.71; LP–126.71: RGA seeding 1–129.44 and RGA seeding 17–128.8). It is evident that the EA method is not so accurate for least cost feed formulation because it uses only mutation as a parameter to improve the diversity of the population in every generation. EA is heuristic in nature but uses only mutation as one parameter to improve the diversity of the problem. Hence, while solving the problem the constraints are not satisfied properly and almost all the constraints are violated. If we do not seed the random number, then we get the wide ranges of solutions in every run most of the time, but unfortunately in this study we did not achieve the optimal solution using EA in MS Excel Solver due to the rigidity of the constraints.

An RGA with seeding technique is developed to overcome the limitation of EA. RGA is also a heuristic technique which works on the principle of the survival of best fit and tournament selection. Adaptive feasibility mutation and heuristic crossover is used along with elitism to solve the LP model for Cattle-1, 2 and 3. Though the seeding technique gives near-optimal answers, we prefer to provide the wide ranges of solutions to farmers in which the values of feedstuffs change in every run where all the constraints will satisfy. As a farmer needs a total mixed ration to feed the cattle on as fresh basis, we have converted the least cost and total mixed ration obtained by all techniques to as fresh basis, and the results are given in Tables 5.5, 5.7 and 5.9. As per the fitment in Table 5.4, an animal of each category requires about 16.75 kg of dry matter from various feed ingredients, which should contain 1644 g of protein, 8542 g of TDN, 117.6 g of calcium and 42 g of phosphorus, and these nutrients can be met from 12.29 kg of roughages and 4.464 kg of concentrate on dry matter. The corresponding TMR cost on dry matter basis is Rs 126.70, that is, Rs 7.56 per kg. As fresh basis is a feed nutrient content with moisture included. After converting to as fresh basis, the feedstuff requirement for Cattle-1 is approximately 30 kg/day, amounting to Rs 5.83/kg using the GRG nonlinear and simplex LP technique. When the expected nutrient requirements were tested using an RGA without seeding and with seeding (RGA1 and RGA17), the least cost ration obtained was Rs 6.05/kg, Rs 5.96/kg and Rs 5.99/kg, respectively. The detailed analysis of rations showed (in Tables 5.4 and 5.5) that this method exactly met the requirement of dry matter, TDN, CP, calcium and phosphorus, and roughage–concentrate was also well within the permissible range. Similar analysis has been done for Cattle-2 (see Tables 5.6 and 5.7), where the least cost ration obtained by various techniques for as fresh basis is Rs 6.08, Rs 6.25, Rs 6.40 and Rs 7.20 per kg by LP simplex, GRG nonlinear, RGA (1) and RGA (17), respectively. For Cattle-3 (see Tables 5.8 and 5.9), the TMR cost for as fresh basis turns out to be Rs 6.38, Rs 6.59, Rs 6.50, Rs 6.50 per kg, respectively. Table 5.10 shows the net profit that farmers can make per cattle in Indian rupees for 10 litres of milk each day on as fresh basis by all techniques. A one-way ANOVA test at 5% level of significance has been performed for the "Null hypothesis: there is no significant difference between techniques". The test reveals that since the P value is greater than 0.05, there is no significance difference between the techniques. Hence, it is proved that the real coded genetic algorithm (RGA) method can be used for ration formulation to find least cost feedstuffs in dairy cattle.

A further linear model was converted to formulate the goal programming model with priority functions. By applying the GP model in this study, the cost of rations could be reduced to a reasonable extent satisfying the exact nutrient requirement. The cost of diet can be reduced by giving first priority to underachievement of least cost and the other priority to overachievement of other nutrients such as CP, TDN, Ca, P, concentrates and roughages on a dry matter basis. Basically, many researchers will try to adjust the dry matter level or change the ratio of concentrates–roughage to reduce the cost of diet by using the GP model, but we have used the same range for constraints which was used earlier for the LP model. Table 5.11 shows the result obtained for GP Model-1, 2 and 3 by the real coded genetic algorithm after assigning the weights on P_1 (goal 1: cost), P_2 (goal 2: CP), P_3 (goal 3: TDN), P_4 (goal 4: Ca), P_5 (goal 5: P), P_6 (goal 6: roughage) and P_7 (goal 7: concentrate) as 0.9, 0.8, 0.7, 0.6, 0.5, 0.4 and 0.3. The results obtained reveal that for GP Model-1, using RGA with hybrid function, we obtain $d_{cost}{}^- = 9.7909$, $d_{TDN}{}^+ = 1.9453$, $d_{Ca}{}^- = 0.0086$, $d_{Ph}{}^- = 0.0132$, $d_{Rough}{}^- = 0.0056$, $d_{Conc}{}^- = 0.0074$ and the rest of the variables $d_{cost}{}^+$, $d_{CP}{}^+$, $d_{CP}{}^-$, $d_{TDN}{}^-$, $d_{Ca}{}^+$, $d_{Ph}{}^+$, $d_{Rough}{}^+$, $d_{Conc}{}^+$ as zero. Goals-1, 4, 5, 6 and7 are overachieved and goal-3 is underachieved, while goal-2 is fully achieved without any deviation, obtaining minimum $(Z) = 0.0127$, which results in a cost of Rs 116.9191/- per kg, per cattle. For GP Model-2, the deviational values are $d_{CP}{}^- = 10.5312$, $d_{CP}{}^- = 0.0002$, $d_{TDN}{}^+ = 1.9789$, $d_{Ca}{}^- = 0.0115$, $d_{Ph}{}^- = 0.011$, $d_{Rough}{}^- = 0.0062$, $d_{Conc}{}^- = 0.0081$, and the rest of the variables $d_{cost}{}^+$, $d_{CP}{}^+$, $d_{TDN}{}^-$, $d_{Ca}{}^+$, $d_{Ph}{}^+$, $d_{Rough}{}^+$, $d_{Conc}{}^+$ as zero, where goals-1, 4, 5, 6 and7 are overachieved and goal-3 is underachieved, while goal-2 is slightly overachieved with $d_{CP}{}^- = 0.0002$ obtaining minimum $(Z) = 0.0132$, amounting to Rs 121.2922/- per kg, per cattle on DM basis. For GP Model-3, the deviational values are $d_{CP}{}^- = 11.4146$, $d_{CP}{}^- = 0.0001$, $d_{TDN}{}^+ = 2.012$, $d_{Ca}{}^- = 0.01$, $d_{Ph}{}^- = 0.0096$, $d_{Rough}{}^- = 0.0054$, $d_{Conc}{}^- = 0.0071$ and the rest of the variables $d_{cost}{}^+$, $d_{CP}{}^+$, $d_{TDN}{}^-$, $d_{Ca}{}^+$, $d_{Ph}{}^+$, $d_{Rough}{}^+$, $d_{Conc}{}^+$ as zero where goals-1, 5, 6 and7 are overachieved and goal-3 is underachieved, while goals-2 and 4 are slightly overachieved with deviation $d_{CP}{}^- = 0.0001$ and $d_{Ca}{}^- = 0.01$ with minimum $(Z) = 0.0115$, amounting to Rs 125.2354/- per kg, per cattle on DM basis. Overall, the cost of Cattle-1, 2 and 3 obtained by the goal programming approach is cheaper by 7.72% for Cattle-1, 7.98% for Cattle-2 and 8.34% for Cattle-3 in comparison with the results obtained by LP model-1, 2 and 3 on dry matter basis, respectively.

The results obtained by the GP model do not completely satisfy the decision maker; therefore, the decision maker needs to work on the overachieved targets. First, the third, fourth, fifth, sixth and seventh goals are analysed, and the reason for the overachievement can be searched for in the diet plan. All possibilities are not considered, as the LP model developed earlier allows the introduction of additional constraints anytime, which results in a new set of solutions, while some constraints (if added) can also lead to "no solution", which means that additional constraints are too complex and it is necessary to mediate in the model by increasing some of the requirements. However, for better output, we need a further discussion with a qualified cattle nutritionist.

Further, in Chapter 6, three goal programming models for non-pregnant buffalo weighing 450 kg and yielding 10 litres of milk with 6% fat are developed on a dry matter basis. In GP Model-1, all eight goals are considered for minimization. In GP Model-2, only two goals, least cost and dry matter, are considered for minimization, and in GP Model-3, other than least cost, all other goals are of a maximizing nature. These GP models are solved by an RGA with the hybrid function "fmincon", and the results obtained reveal that an RHGA can effectively be used to economize the total mixed ration cost such that the feed requirements of the animals are met without any nutrient deficiency. Initially, the linear model is considered and solved by real coded GA with different parameters, and due to the large dimension of the problem and rigidity in constraints, we opted to develop an RHGA to solve the ration formulation problem for buffaloes. This category of animal requires 16.42 kg of dry matter from various kinds of feedstuffs, which should contain 1715.8 g of protein, 9183.5 g of TDN, 74.8 g of calcium and 40.5 g of phosphorus. As per the LP model solved using hybrid GA, this requirement can be met from 13.13 kg of roughage and 3.28 kg of concentrates on dry matter. Its corresponding cost on dry matter basis is Rs 101.6703/- per kg, per buffalo. As fresh basis is a feed nutrient content with moisture included for total mixed ration (TMR); hence, it requires approximately 36.3 kg TMR, amounting to Rs 4.5/- per kg. By GP Model-1 the approximately cost of ration is Rs 100.7965/-on DM basis, which corresponds to 26.9 kg TMR, amounting to Rs 5.01/- per Kg, where the goals 1, 2 3, 4, 6 and 7 are overachieved and goals 5 and 7 are fully achieved. This GP model corresponds to least cost, but the constraints such as least cost, CP, TDN, P, roughage and concentrates are decreased by 14%, 17.4%, 16.5%, 29.13% and 17.594%, and calcium and phosphorus are achieved completely, 100%. Therefore, to overcome this deficiency, GP Model-2 is formulated with only two priority goals (minimizing least cost and DMI), and the results obtained revealed that all the goals are completely achieved with least cost of Rs 101.6090/- on DM basis, which leads to approximately 30 kg of TMR, amounting to Rs 4.7/- per kg. Goals 1 and 2 are fully achieved, and remaining goals are either underachieved or overachieved. GP Model-3 is also formulated with the objective of minimizing the cost of the ration by not considering dry matter as a goal in the objective function. Dry matter is treated as a constraint directly, from which we observe that on assigning the weights P_1 (goal 1: cost), P_2 (goal 2: CP), P_3 (goal 3: TDN), P_4 (goal 4: Ca), P_5 (goal 5: P), P_6 (goal 6: roughage), P_7 (goal 7: concentrate) as 0.9, 0.8, 0.7, 0.6, 0.5, 0.4 and 0.3 and solving the GP Model using RGA with hybrid function, we obtain: $d_{cost}^- = 0.0021$, $d_{CP}^+ = 0.4508$, $d_{TDN}^+ = 0.0901$, $d_{Ca}^+ = 0.9891$, $d_{Ph}^+ = 0.0499$, and the rest of the deviational variables d_{cost}^+, d_{CP}^-, d_{TDN}^-, d_{Ca}^-, d_{Ph}^-, d_{Rough}^-, d_{Rough}^+, d_{Conc}^-, d_{Conc}^+ are zero. We observe that goal 1 is overachieved; goals 2, 3, 4 and 5 are underachieved, while goals 6 and 7 are fully achieved without any deviation, with a minimum cost of Rs 101.605/- on DM basis. All three GP models give a wide range of solutions, but the obtained result does not completely satisfy the decision maker/nutritionist, as the reasons for underachievement and overachievement targets need to be analysed further, where the choice of a final solution depends upon the decision maker. There is a need for further discussion with a nutritionist for better output.

The results of the study from Chapters 4, 5 and 6 reveal that after keeping the nutritional requirements of dairy cattle and buffalo at different body conditions, the integrated linear and simple goal programming model with weighted priority function was sufficient to optimize the ration cost. The ration cost obtained by this method was reasonably cheaper than when formulated by only the LP approach. The requirement of nutrients (CP, TDN, Ca, P, roughage and concentrates) was met by fine-tuning the individual feedstuffs. The roughage–concentrates and other constraints maximum–minimum range make the model more rigid, and hence the binary coded genetic algorithm was not suggested to solve the problem. To overcome the limitation of the binary genetic algorithm, it was also proved that the use of the RGA is a better technique for a good quality feed mix to dairy cattle for better health and milk production over other conventional methods, viz. LP simplex, GRG nonlinear and EA and hence can also be used for ration formulation to find least cost feedstuffs in dairy cattle. All the techniques – viz. RGA without crossover, RGA without mutation, RGA with crossover and mutation and RGA with hybrid function – for least cost ration perform equally. RGA without crossover and RGA without mutation provide near-optimal answers, but solutions seem to get stuck in local minima; hence, it is proved that RGA with a hybrid function provides the optimal solution, and this method can also be used for a ration formulation to find least cost feedstuffs for dairy buffalo.

References

19 Livestock Census–2012. *All India Report Ministry of Agriculture Department of Animal Husbandry*. New Delhi: Dairying and Fisheries Krishi Bhavan.

Afolayan, M., Olatunde, A. M. and Afolayan, M. 2008. 'Nigeria Oriented Poultry Feed Formulation Software Requirements'. *Journal of Applied Sciences Research*. Vol. 4. Pp. 1596–1602.

Afrouziyeh, M., Shivazad, M., Chamani, M. and Dashti, G. 2010. 'Use of Non-linear Programming to Determine the Economically Optimal Energy Density in Laying Hens' Diet During Phase 1'. *African Journal of Agricultural Research*. Vol. 5. Pp. 2270–2777.

Al-Deseit, B. 2009. 'Least-Cost Broiler Ration Formulation Using Linear Programming Technique'. *Journal of Animal and Veterinary Advances*. Vol. 8. Pp. 1274–1278.

Aletor, V. A. 1986. 'Some Agro-Industrial By-products and Wastes in Livestock Feeding: A Review of Prospects and Problems'. *World Review of Animal Production*. Vol. 22. Pp. 35–41.

Ali, M. A. and Leeson, S. 1995. 'The Nutritive Value of Some Indigenous Asian Poultry Feed Ingredients'. *Animal Feed Science and Technology*. Vol. 55. Pp. 227–237.

Almasad, M., Altahat, A. and Al-Sharafat, A. 2011. 'Applying Linear Programming Technique to Formulate Least Cost Balanced Ration for White Egg Layers in Jordan'. *International Journal of Empirical Research*. Vol. 1. Pp. 112–120.

Angadi, U. B., Anandan, S., Gowda, N. K. S., Rajendran, D., Devi, L., Elangovan, A. V. and Jash, S. 2016. '"Feed Assis" – An Expert System on Balanced Feeding for Dairy Animals'. *AGRIS On-line Papers in Economics and Informatics*. Vol. 8(3). Pp. 3–12.

Annual Report. 2016. *Department of Animal Husbandry, Dairying and Fisheries, Ministry of Agriculture and Farmers Welfare*. Govt. of India.

Babic, Z. and Peric, T. 2011. 'Optimization of Livestock Feed Blend by Use of Goal Programming'. *International Journal of Production Economics*. Vol. 130. Pp. 218–223.

Bajpai, P. and Kumar, M. 2010. 'Genetic Algorithm—an Approach to Solve Global Optimization Problems'. *Indian Journal of Computer Science and Engineering*. Vol. 1(3). Pp. 199–206.

Baron, L., Achiche, S. and Balazinski, M. 2002. 'Fuzzy Decisions Systemknowledge Base Generation Using a Genetic Algorithm'. *International Journal of Approximate Reasoning*. Vol. 28. Pp. 125–148.

Basic Animal Husbandry & Fisheries Statistics. 2017. AHS Series-18. New Delhi: Government of India Ministry of Agriculture & Farmers Welfare Department of Animal Husbandry. Dairying and Fisheries Krishi Bhavan.

Bath, D. L. 1985. 'Nutritional Requirements and Economics of Lowering Feed Costs'. *Journal of Dairy Science*. Vol. 68(6). Pp. 1579–1584.

Bharti. 1993. 'Controlled Random Search Optimization Techniques and Their Applications'. Ph.D. Thesis. India: U.O.R. Roorkee.

Biggs, M. C. 1975. 'Constrained Minimization Using Recursive Quadratic Programming'. In *Towards Global Optimization* (L. C. W. Dixon and G. P. Szergo, eds.). North Holland. Pp. 341–349.

Black, J. R. and Hlubik, J. 1980. 'Basics of Computerized Linear Programs for Ration Formulation'. *Journal of Dairy Science*. Vol. 63. Pp. 1366–1377.

Bremermann, H. J. and Anderson, R. W. 1989. 'An Alternative to Backpropagation: A Simple Rule of Synaptic Modification for Neural Net Training and Memory'. Technical Report: U.C. Berkeley Center for Pure and Applied Mathematics PAM-483.

Brooks, S. H. 1958. 'A Discussion of Random Methods for Seeking Maxima.' *Operations Research*. Vol. 6. Pp. 244–251.

Broyden, C. G. 1967. 'Quasi-Newton Methods and Their Application to Function Minimization'. *Mathemutics of Computation*. Vol. 21. Pp. 368–381.

Castrodeza, C., Lara, P. and Pen, T. 2005. 'Multicriteria Fractional Model for Feed Formulation: Economic, Nutritional and Environmental Criteria'. *Agricultural Systems*. Vol. 86. Pp. 76–96.

Chakeredza, S., Akinnifesi, F. K., Ajayi, O. C., Sileshi, G., Mngomba, S. and Gondwe, F. M. T. 2008. 'A Simple Method of Formulating Least-cost Diets for Smallholder Dairy Production in Sub-sub-Saharan Africa'. *African Journal of Biotechnology*. Vol. 7. Pp. 2925–2933.

Chavas, J.-P., Kliebenstein, J. and Crenshaw, T. 'Modeling Dynarnic (August 1985): Agricultural Production Response: The Case of Swine Production.' *American Journal of Agricultural Economics*. Vol. 67. Pp. 636–646.

Clark, J. H. and Davis, C. L. 1980. 'Some Aspects of Feeding High Producing Dairy Cows'. *Journal of Dairy Science*. Vol. 63. P. 873.

Dantzig, G. B. 1951. 'Application of the Simplex Method to a Transportation Problem', *Activity Analysis of Production and Allocation*. Koopmans, T.C., Ed., John Wiley and Sons, New York, Pp. 359–373.

Dantzig, G. B. 1963. *Linear Programming and Extension*. Princeton, NJ: Princeton University Press and the Rand Corporation.

Davies, D. 1970. 'Some Practical Methods of Optimization'. In *Integer and Nonlinear Programming* (J. Abadie ed.), North-Holland Publishing Co., Amsterdam, 1970.

Davis, L. 1989. 'Adapting Operator Probabilities in Genetic Algorithms'. In *Proceedings of the Third International Conference on Genetic Algorithms* (J. David Schaer ed.). San Mateo: Morgan Kaufmann Publishers). Pp. 61–69.

Deb, K. 1999. 'An Introduction to Genetic Algorithms'. *Sadhana*. Vol. 24. Pp. 293–315. Doi: https://doi.org/10.1007/BF02823145.

Deb, K. 2009. *Optimization for Engineering Design*; 2010, PHI. ISBN-978-81-203-0943-2.

Dent, J. B. and Casey, H. 1967. *Linear Programming and Animal Nutrition*. London: Crosby Lockwood.

Dixon, L. C. W. 1972a. *Nonlinear Optimization*. London: English Universities Press.

Dixon, L. C. W. 1972b. 'Variable Metric Algorithms: Necessary and Sufficient Conditions for Identical Behavior of Nonquadratic Functions'. *Journal of Optimization Theory and Applications*. Vol. 10. Pp. 34–40.

Dixon, L. C. W. 1973a. 'ACSIM: An Accelerated Constrained Simplex Technique'. *ComputerAided Design*. Vol. 5. Pp. 23–32.

Dixon, L. C. W. 1973b. 'Conjugate Directions Without Line Searches'. *Journal of the Institute of Mathematics Applications*. Vol. 11. Pp. 317–328.

Dixon, L. C. W. (ed.). 1976. *Optimization in Action*. New York: Academic Press.

Eila, N., Lavvaf, A. and Farahvash, T. 2012. 'A Model for Obtaining More Economic Diets for Laying Hen'. *African Journal of Agricultural Research*. Vol. 7(8). Pp. 1302–1306.

Fletcher, R. 1987. *Practical Methods of Optimization*. John Wiley and Sons. The Atrium, Southern Gate, Chichester, ISBN: 9780471915478.

Furuya, T., Satake, T. and Minami, Y. 1997. 'Evolutionary Programming for Mix Design'. *Computers and Electronics in Agriculture*. Vol. 18(3). Pp. 129–135.

Gale, D., Kuhn, H. W. and Tucker, A. W. 1951. 'Linear Programming and the Theory of Games'. In *Activity Analysis of Production and Allocation* (T. C. Koopmans ed.). New York: Wiley & Sons, Pp. 317–335.

Gallenti, G. 1997. The Use of Computer for the Analysis of Input Demand in Farm Management: A Multicriteria Approach to the Diet Problem. First European Conference for Information Technology in Agriculture, 15–18 June 1997.

Garg, M. R., FAO. 2012. 'Balanced Feeding for Improving Livestock Productivity— Increase in Milk Production and Nutrient use Efficiency and Decrease in Methane Emission'. *FAO Animal Production and Health, Paper No. 173*. Rome, Italy.

Garg, M. R., Sherasia, P. L., Bhanderi, B. M. and Makkar, H. P. S. 2016. 'Nitrogen Use Efficiency for Milk Production on Feeding a Balanced Ration and Predicting Manure Nitrogen Excretion in Lactating Cows and Buffaloes Under Tropical Conditions'. *Animal Nutrition and Feed Technology*. Vol. 16. Pp. 1–12.

Gen, M. and Cheng, R. 1997. *Genetic Algorithm and Engineering Design*. New York: John Wiley and Son. ISBN: 0-471-12741-8.

Ghosh, S., Ghosh, J., Pal, D. T. and Gupta, R. 2014. 'Current Concepts of Feed Formulation for Livestock using Mathematical Modeling'. *Animal Nutrition and Feed Technology*. Vol. 14. Pp. 205–223.

Gill, P. E., Murray, W. and Wright, M. H. 1981. *Practical Optimization*. London: Academic Press.

Goldberg, D. E. 1989. *Genetic Algorithms in Search, Optimization, and Machine Learning*. Reading, MA: Addison-Wesley.

Goldfarb, D. 1969a. 'Extension of Davidon's Variable Metric Method to Maximization Under Linear Inequality and Equality Constraints'. *SIAM Journal on Applied Mathematics*. Vol. 17. Pp. 739–764.

Gosh, S. 2011, September. 'Least Cost Ration Formulation in Animal Using Mathematical Modeling: An Integrated Linear and Weighted Goal Programming Approach'. Unpublished M.Phil. Dissertation. Jain University.

Govt of India. 2012. *Ministry of Agriculture Department of Animal Husbandry*. New Delhi: Dairying and fisheries Krishi Bhavan, 19 livestock census all India report.

Guevara, V. R. 2004. 'Use of Nonlinear Programming to Optimize Performance Response to Energy Density in Broiler Feed Formulation'. *Poultry Science*. Vol. 83(2). Pp. 147–151.

Gupta, R. and Chandan, M. 2013. 'Use of Controlled Random Search Technique for Global Optimization" in Animal Diet Problem'. *International Journal of Emerging Technology and Advanced Engineering*. Vol. 3(2).

Gupta, R., Chandan, M. and Kuntal, R. S. 2013a. 'Heuristic Approaches in Solving Non-Linear Programming Model of Livestock Ration for Global Optimization'. *International Journal of Engineering Sciences and Emerging Technologies (IJESET)*. Vol. 6(1). Pp. 37–48.

Gupta, R., Kuntal, R. S. and Ramesh, K. 2013b. 'Heuristic Approach to Goal Programming Problem for Animal Ration Formulation'. *International Journal of Engineering and Innovative Technology (IJEIT)*. Vol. 3(4). Pp. 414–422.

Haar, V. and M. J. Black. 1991. 'Ration Formulation Using Linear Programming'. *Veterinary Clinics of North America: Food Animal Practice*. Vol. 7. Pp. 541–556.

Hadrich, J. C., Wolf, C. A., Black, J. R. and Harsh, S. B. 2008. 'Incorporating Environmentally Compliant Manure Nutrient Disposal Costs into Least-Cost Livestock Ration Formulation'. *Journal of Agricultural and Applied Economics*. Vol. 40(1). Pp. 287–300.

Han, S. P. 1977. 'A Globally Convergent Method for Nonlinear Programming'. *Journal of Optimization Theory and Applications*. Vol. 22. P. 297.

Herrera, F., Lozano, M. and Verdegay, J. L. 1995. 'Fuzzy Connective based Crossover Operators to Model Genetic Algorithms Population Diversity. Technical Report No. DECSAI-95110, University of Granada, 18071 Granada, Spain.

Hertzler, G. 1987. 'Dynamically Optimal and Approximately Optimal Beef Cattle Diets Formulated by Nonlinear Programming'. *Western Journal of Agricultural Economics*. Vol. 13. Pp. 7–17.

Hertzler, G. 1988. 'Dynamically Optimal and Approximately Optimal Beef Cattle Diets Formulated by Nonlinear Programming'. *Western Journal of Agricultural Economics*. Vol. 13(1). Pp. 7–17.

Himmelblau, D. M. 1972. *Applied Nonlinear Programming*. New York: McGraw-Hill.

Hock, W. and Schittkowski, K. 1983. 'A Comparative Performance Evaluation of 27 Nonlinear Programming Codes'. *Computing*. Vol. 30. Pp. 335–358.

Holland, J. H. 1975. *Adaptation in Natural and Artificial Systems*. Ann Arbor, MI: University of Michigan Press.

Jean dit Bailleul, P., Rivest, J., Dubeau, F. and Pomar, C. 2001. 'Reducing Nitrogen Excretion in Pigs by Modifying the Traditional Least-cost Formulation Algorithm'. *Livestock Production Science*. Vol. 72. Pp. 199–211.

Koda, M. 2012. 'Chaos Search in Fourier Amplitude Sensitivity Test Version'. *Journal of Information and Communication Technology*. Vol. 11. Pp. 1–16.

Kumar, J. R. K. 2012. 'Effect of Polygamy with Selection in Genetic Algorithm'. *International Journal of Soft Computing and Engineering*. Vol. 2(1). ISSN: 2231-2307.

Kuntal R.S., Gupta R., Rajendran D., Patil V. 2019. 'Study of Real-Coded Hybrid Genetic Algorithm (RGA) to Find Least-Cost Ration for Non-Pregnant Dairy Buffaloes'. In: J. C. Bansal, K. N. Das, A. Nagar, K. Deep, A. K. Ojha (Eds.), *Intelligent Systems and Computing 817: Soft Computing for Problem Solving, Springer Nature Singapore Pte Ltd.,* Pp.369–389. ISBN: 9789811315947.

Kuntal, R. S., Gupta, R., Rajendran, D. and Patil, V. 2016. 'Application of Real Coded Genetic Algorithm (RGA) to Find Least Cost Feedstuffs for Dairy Cattle During Pregnancy'. *Asian Journal of Animal and Veterinary Advances*. Vol. 11. Pp. 594–607.

Kuntal, R. S., Gupta, R., Rajendran, D. and Patil, V. 2018. 'A Goal Programming Approach to Ration Formulation Problem for Indian Dairy Cows'. *International Journal of Current Advanced Research*. Vol. 7(4c). Pp. 11506–11510.

Lara, P. 1993. 'Multiple Objective Fractional Programming and Livestock Ration Formulation: A Case Study for Dairy Cow Diets in Spain'. *Agricultural Systems.* Vol. 41. Pp. 321–334.

Leng, R. A. 1991. 'Feeding Strategies for Improving Milk Production of Dairy Animals Managed by Small Holder Farmers in the Tropics,' L. Speedy, A., Sansoucy, R. (Eds.), *Feeding Dairy Cows in the Tropics, FAO, Rome.* Pp. 82–104.

Lucasius, C. B. and Kateman, G. 1989. 'Applications of Genetic Algorithms in Chemometrics'. In *Proceedings ofthe 3rd International Conference on Genetic Algorithms.* Morgan Kaufmann, Los Altos, CA. Pp. 170–176.

MacDonald, Z. 1995. 'Teaching Linear Programming using Microsoft Excel Solver'. *Computers in Higher Education Economics Review.* Vol. 9(3). Pp. 7–10.

McCormick, G. P. 1970. 'The Variable Reduction Method for Nonlinear Programming'. *Management Science Theory.* Vol. 17. Pp. 146–160.

McCormick, G. P. 1983. *Nonlinear Programming: Theory, Algorithms, and Applications.* New York: Wiley, P. 444.

Meyer, J. H. and W. N. Garrett. 1967. 'Efficiency of Feed Utilization'. *Journal of Animal Science.* Vol. 26. P. 638.

Meyer, K. 1985. 'Genetic Parameters of Dairy Production of Australian Black and White Cows'. *Livestock Production Science.* Vol. 12. P. 205.

Mitani, K. and Nakayama, H. 1997. 'A Multi-objective Diet Planning Support System Using the Satisfying Trade-off Method'. *Journal of Multi-Criteria Decision Analysis.* Vol. 6. Pp. 131–139.

Mohan, C. and Shanker, K. 1994. 'A Random Search Technique for Global optimization Based on Quadratic Approximation'. *Asia Pacific Journal of Operations Research.* Vol. 11. Pp. 93–101.

Mondal, M. S., Yamaguchi, H., Date, Y., Shimbara, T., Toshinai, K., Shimomura, Y., Mori, M. and Nakazato, M. 2003. 'A Role for Neuropeptide W in the Regulation of Feeding Behavior'. *Endocrinology.* Vol. 144(11,1). Pp. 4729–4733. https://doi.org/10.1210/en.2003-0536

Mudgal, V., Mehta, M. K., Rane, A. S. and Nanavati, S. 2003. 'A Survey on Feeding Practices and Nutritional Status of Dairy Animals in Madhya Pradesh'. *Indian Journal of Animal Nutrition.* Vol. 20(2). Pp. 217–220.

Munford, A. G. 1989. 'A Microcomputer System for Formulating Animal Diets Which May Involve Liquid Raw Materials'. *European Journal of Operational Research.* Vol. 41. Pp. 270–276.

Munford, A. G. 1996. 'The Use of Iterative Linear Programming in Practical Applications of Animal Diet Formulation'. *Mathematics and Computers in Simulation.* Vol. 42. Pp. 255–261.

Munford, A. G. 2005. The Ultramix-Professional Feed Formulation and Livestock Modelling System. Udine, Italy: AGM Systems Ltd.

Nabasirye, M., Mugisha, J. V. T., Tibayungwa, F. and Kyarisiima, C. C. 2011. 'Optimization of Input in Animal Production: A Linear Programming Approach to the Ration Formulation Problem'. *International Research Journal of Agricultural Science and Soil Science* (ISSN: 2251–0044). Vol. 1(7). Pp. 22:1–226.

National Research Council. 1981. *Effect of Environment on Nutrient Requirements of Domestic Animals.* Washington, DC: The National Academies Press.

National Research Council. 2001. *Nutrient Requirements of Dairy Cattle* (7th rev. ed.). Washington, DC: National Academic Science.

Nocedal, J. and Wright, S. J. 2006. *Numerical Optimization*. Second edition. Springer Series in Operations Research. Springer Verlag. Springer Science+Business Media, LLC. ISBN-10: 0-387-30303-0.

Nott, H. and Combs, G. F. 1967. 'Data Processing Feed Ingredient Composition Data'. *Feedstuffs*. Vol. 39. Pp. 21–22.

Nutrient Requirements of Animals-Cattle and Buffalo (ICAR-NIANP). 2013. ISBN: 978-81-7164-139-9.

Oladokun, V. O. and Johnson, A. 2012. 'Feed Formulation in Nigerian Poultry Farms: A Mathematical Programming Approach'. *American Journal of Scientific and Industrial Research*. Vol. 3. Pp. 14–20.

Olorunfemi, T. O. S., Aderibigbe, F. M., Falaki, S. O., Adebayo, O. T. and Fasakin, E. A. 2001. 'An Overview of Linear Programming Application to Least-cost Ration Formulation in Aquaculture'. *Journal of Technology and Science*. Vol. 5. Pp. 84–92.

Olson, D. L. and Swenseth, S. R. 1987. 'A Linear Approximation for Chance-Constrained Programming'. *Journal of the Operational Research Society*. Vol. 38(3). Pp. 261–267.

Ono, I., Kita, H. and Kobayashi, S. 2003. 'A Real-coded Genetic Algorithm using the Unimodal Normal Distribution Crossover'. In *Advances in Evolutionary Computing* (A. Ghosh and S. Tsutsui, eds.). Natural Computing Series. Berlin, Heidelberg: Springer. https://doi.org/10.1007/978-3-642-18965-4_8

Panne, C. V. D. and Popp, W. 1963. 'Minimum-cost Cattle Feed Under Probabilistic Protein Constraints'. *Management Science*. Vol. 9. Pp. 405–430.

Patrick, H. and Schaible, P. J. 1980. *Poultry: Feed and Nutrition* (2nd Edn.), AVI Publishing, USA. Pp: 417–458.

Pesti, G. M. and Siela, A. F. 1999. 'The Use of an Electronic Spreadsheet to Solve Linear and Non-linear "Stochastic" Feed Formulation Problems'. *Journal of Applied Poultry Research*. Vol. 8. Pp. 110–121.

Pond, W. G., Church, D. C. and Pond, K. R. 1995. *Basic Animal Nutrition and Feeding*. Canada: John Wiley and Sons, Inc.

Powell, M. J. D. 1977. 'Quadratic Termination Properties of Davidon's New Variable Metric Algorithm'. *Mathematical Programming*. Vol. 12. Pp. 141–147.

Powell, M. J. D. 1978a. 'The Convergence of Variable Metric Methods for Nonlinearly Constrained Optimization Calculations'. In *Nonlinear Programming 3*, (O. L. Mangasarian, R. R. Meyer and S. M. Robinson, eds.). Academic Press, New York.

Powell, M. J. D. 1978b. 'A Fast Algorithm for Nonlinearly Constrained Optimization Calculations'. In *Numerical Analysis*. Vol. 630 (G. A. Watson, ed.). Lecture Notes in Mathematics. Springer Verlag, Berlin.

Pratiksha, S. 2011. Optimization Techniques for Animal Diet Formulation, Gate2Biotech, e-portal, February 2011, Vol. 1(2). Pp. 1–5, ISSN 1802-2685, Europe.

Radhika, V. and Rao, S. B. N. 2010. 'Formulation of Low-cost Balanced Ration for Livestock Using Microsoft Excel'. *Wayamba Journal of Animal Science*. Pp. 38–41.

Ranjan, S. K. 1998. *Nutrient Requirements of Livestock and Poultry*. New Delhi: Indian Council of Agricultural Research.

Reddy, A. A., Rani, C. R., Cadman, T., Kumar, S. N. and Reddy, A. N. 2016. 'Towards Sustainable Indicators of Food and Nutritional Outcomes in India. *World Journal of Science, Technology and Sustainable Development*. Vol. 13(2). Pp. 128–142. https://doi.org/10.1108/WJSTSD-10-2015-0049

Rehman, A. R. 2014. 'Evolutionary Algorithms with Average Crossover and Power Heuristics for Aquaculture Diet Formulation'. Ph.D. Thesis. Sintok, Malaysia: University Utara Malaysia.

Rehman, T. and Romero, C. 1984. 'Multiple-criteria Decision-making Techniques and Their Role in Livestock Ration Formulation'. *Agricultural Systems*. Vol. 15. Pp. 23–49.

Rehman, T. and Romero, C. 1987. 'Goal Programming with Penalty Functions and Livestock Ration Formulation'. *Agricultural Systems*. Vol. 23. Pp. 117–132.

Romero, C. and Rehman, T. 1984. Goal Programming and Multiple Criteria Decision-making in Farm Planning: An Expository Analysis. *Journal of Agricultural Economics*. Vol. 35. Pp. 177–190. doi:10.1111/J.1477-9552.1984.TB02045.X.

Rose, S. P. 1997. *Principles of Poultry Science*. CAB International, Wallingford, Oxon, ISBN: 0 85199 122X.

Rossi, R. 2004. 'Least-cost Formulation Software: An Introduction'. *Aqua Feed Formul Beyond*. Vol. 3. Pp. 3–5.

Roush, W. B., Stock, R. H., Cravener, T. L. and D'Alfonso, T. H. 1994. 'Using Chance-Constrained Programming for Animal Feed Formulation at Agway'. *Interfaces*. Vol. 24(2). Pp. 53–58.

Şahman, M. A., Çunkaş, M., İnal, Ş., İnal, F., Coşkun, B. and Taşkiran, U. 2009. 'Cost Optimization of Feed Mixes by Genetic Algorithms'. *Advances in Engineering Software*. Vol. 40(10). Pp. 965–974.

Saxena, P. 2011a. 'Comparison of Linear and Non-linear Programming Techniques for Animal Diet'. *Applied Mathematics*. Vol. 1(2). Pp. 106–108. https://doi.org/10.5923/j.am.20110102.17

Saxena, P. 2011b. 'Application of Nonlinear Programming for Optimization of Nutrient Requirements for Maximum Weight Gain in Buffaloes'. *International Journal of Food Science and Nutrition Engineering*. Vol. 1(1). Pp. 8–10.

Saxena, P. 2011c. 'Optimization Techniques for Animal Diet Formulation'. *www. Gate2Biotech.com*. Vol. 1(2). Pp. 1–5.

Sebastian, C., Akinnifesi, F. K., Ajayi, O., Sileshi, G., Mngomba, S. and Gondwe, F. M. T. 2008. 'A Simple Method of Formulating Least-cost Diets for Smallholder Dairy Production in Sub-Saharan Africa'. *African Journal of Biotechnology*. Vol. 7. Pp. 2925–2933.

Shilpa, J., Dinesh, B. and Prakash, C. 2013. 'Comparative Analysis of Real and Binary Coded Genetic Algorithm for Fuzzy Time Series Prediction'. *International Journal of Education and Information Sciences*, Vol. 3. Pp. 299–304.

Singh, K. P. and Singh, I. 2015. 'Buffalo Diversity in India: Breeds and Defined Populations'. *Dairy Year Book*. (2014–15) Pp. 33–36.

Sklan, D. and Dariel, I. 1993. 'Diet Planning for Humans Using Mixed-integer Linear Programming'. *British Journal of Nutrition*. Vol. 70. Pp. 27–35.

Taha, H.A. 1987. *Operations Research* (4th Edn.). United States edition: Macmillan Publishing Co. P. 876.

Tedeschi, L. O., Fox, D. G., Chase, L. E. and Wang, S. J. 2004. 'Whole-herd Optimization with the CornellNet Carbohydrate and Protein System: Predicting Feed Biological Values for Diet Optimization Withlinear Programming'. *Poultry Science*. Vol. 83. Pp. 147–151.

Tedeschi, L. O., Fox, D. G., Sainz, R. D., Barioni, L. G., de Medeiros, S. R. and Boin, C. 2005. Mathematical Models in Ruminant Nutrition. *Scientia Agricola*. Vol. 62. Pp. 76–91.

Townsley, R. 1968. 'Derivation of Optimal Livestock Rations Using Quadratic Programming. *Journal of Agricultural Economics*. Vol. 19(3). Pp. 347–354.

Tozer, P. R. 2000. 'Least-Cost Ration Formulations for Holstein Dairy Heifers By Using Linear and Stochastic Programming'. *Journal of Dairy Science*. Vol. 83. Pp. 443–451.

Tozer, P. R. and Stokes, J. R. 2001. 'A Multiobjective Programming Approach to Feed Ration Balancing and Nutrient Management'. *Agricultural Systems*. Vol. 67(3). Pp. 201–215.

Van de Panne, C. and Popp, W. 1963. 'Minimum-Cost Cattle Feed Und- er Probabilistic Protein Constarints'. *Management Science*. Vol. 9(3). Pp. 405–430.

Xiong, B-H., Luo, Q-Y. and Pang, Z-H. 2003. Application of Dual Model in Animal Feed Formulation optimization System. *Scientia Agricultura Sinica*. Vol. 2003. Pp. 1347–1351.

Waugh, F. 1951. 'The Minimum-Cost Dairy Feed'. *Journal of Farm Economics*. Vol. 33. Pp. 299–310.

Zgajnar, J., Juvancic, L. and Kavcic, S. 2009. 'Combination of Linear and Weighted Goal Programming with Penalty Function in Optimization of Daily Dairy Cow Ration'. *Agricultural Economics—Czech*. Pp. 492–500.

Zgajnar, J. and Kavcic, S. 2008. 'Spreadsheet Tool for Least-cost and Nutrition Balanced Beef Ration Formulation'. *Acta Agriculturae Slovenia*. Vol. 2(Suppl.). Pp. 187–194.

Zgajnar, J. and Kavcic, S. 2009. 'Multi-goal Pig Ration Formulation; Mathematical Optimization Approach'. *Agronomy Research*. Vol. 7. Pp. 775–782.

Zhang, F. and Roush, W. B. 2002. 'Multiple-objective (Goal) Programming Model for Feed Formulation: An Example for Reducing Nutrient Variation'. *Poultry Science*. Vol. 81. Pp. 182–192.

Zheng, D. W., et al. 1996. 'Evolution Program for Nonlinear Goal Programming'. *18th International Conference on Computers and Industrial Engineering*.

Index

Note: Numbers in **bold** indicate tables and those in *italics* indicate figures.

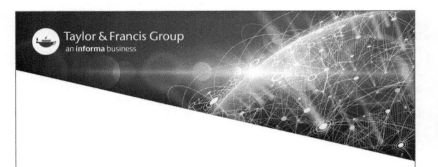

For Product Safety Concerns and Information please contact our EU
representative GPSR@taylorandfrancis.com
Taylor & Francis Verlag GmbH, Kaufingerstraße 24, 80331 München, Germany

www.ingramcontent.com/pod-product-compliance
Ingram Content Group UK Ltd.
Pitfield, Milton Keynes, MK11 3LW, UK
UKHW051941210425
457613UK00026BA/59